RENAL CARE:

Resources And Practical Applications

Kerri L. Wiggins, MS, RD

Renal Dietitians Dietetic Practice Group

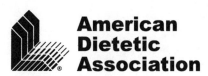

Diana Faulhaber, Publisher
Jason M. Muzinic, Acquisitions Editor
Elizabeth Nishiura, Production Editor

10 9 8 7 6 5 4 3 2 1

Library of Congress Cataloging-in-Publication Data

Wiggins, Kerri Lynn.
    Renal care : resources and practical applications / Kerri L.
Wiggins ; Renal Dietitians Dietetic Practice Group American
Dietetic Association.
        p. ; cm.
Includes index.
    ISBN 0-88091-336-3
    1. Chronic renal failure—Diet therapy.   2. Chronic renal failure
—Patients—Nutrition—Evaluation.   I. American Dietetic Associa-
tion. Renal Practice Group.   II. Title.
    [DNLM: 1. Kidney Failure, Chronic—diet therapy. 2. Nutrition
Assessment.   WJ 342 W655r 2003]
RC918.R4W497 2003
616.6'140654—dc21
                                                         2003012120

Contents

Sections

Acknowledgements

I wish to extend my thanks and appreciation to the following individuals, who provided direction and assistance during the development of this publication. They contributed their time and expertise to ensure that this guide would be of the utmost quality.

Joan Brookhyser, RD, CSR
Betty Fisher, MS, RD
Kathy Schiro Harvey, MS, RD, CSR
Ann Lipkin, MS, RD
Carole McCorry, RD
Katy Wilkens, MS, RD

Reviewers

Barbara A. Bailey, RD
Good Samaritan Hospital Dialysis
Baltimore, Maryland

Laura K. Joseph, MS, RD, CSR
Regional Kidney Centers
Fayetteville, Arkansas

Lisa Murphy, MSEd, RD, CSR
Renal Dietitian
Grand Island, New York

Preface

In 2002 the American Dietetic Association published the 3rd edition of *Guidelines for Nutrition Care of Renal Patients.* That book presents extensive guidelines based on the best available scientific information and expert opinion. During the process of revising the *Guidelines,* the decision was made to expand upon the appendixes that were included in the 2nd edition and place the information in a separate publication, thus providing easier access to the information. This was the foundation for *Renal Care: Resources and Practical Applications.*

This publication is divided into 20 sections, each of which addresses a key factor in the nutrition assessment of individuals with chronic kidney disease (CKD). The sections provide in-depth coverage of the available methods for assessing nutritional status and discuss how these methods relate to the care of individuals with CKD. Formulas and tables are included, allowing the practitioner to find in one location all the information needed to provide the nutrition care outlined in the *Guidelines for Nutrition Care of Renal Patients,* 3rd edition.

This publication was written using the most current scientific literature available. Recommendations from the National Kidney Foundation's Kidney Disease Outcomes Quality Initiative (K/DOQI) Guidelines have been included in many of the sections. It is hoped that this publication will prove to be a valuable resource to those who provide nutrition care to patients with renal disease.

Introduction

The *Guidelines for Nutrition Care of Renal Patients,* 3rd edition, supply a framework for providing nutrition care to individuals with chronic kidney disease (CKD). An important aspect of providing nutrition care is the assessment of nutritional status of the patient. Nutrition assessment involves many factors and is complicated further in individuals with CKD. This publication is comprised of information to aid in the assessment of the individual with CKD, as outlined in the *Guidelines for Nutrition Care of Renal Patients,* 3rd edition.

Twenty sections are presented in this publication. Each discusses a specific topic related to nutrition assessment and considers how the methodology or interpretation of that topic may be altered when assessing the nutrition status of CKD patients. Several sections review the use of anthropometrics in assessing nutritional status; some provide guidelines and formulas for assessing dialysis adequacy and protein balance; and others discuss issues related to CKD that need to be considered when evaluating nutritional status of individuals with CKD. The sections are listed below with brief descriptions of the specifics they contain:

Section 1: Federal Regulations—Reproduces a section of the Code of Federal Regulations that details the minimum requirements for adequate provision of patient care in outpatient dialysis units.

Section 2: Height Determination—Reviews the importance of and procedure for obtaining an accurate height. Provides methods of determining stature from arm span and knee height measurements if a patient is unable to stand.

Section 3: Evaluation of Body Weight—Presents ideal body weight, standard body weight, and body mass index (BMI) and discusses the relative merits and disadvantages of the methods for evaluating weight. Recommends levels of body weight for CKD patients and provides methods for adjusting weight for amputation and obesity.

Section 4: Frame Size Determinations—Details the use of wrist circumference and elbow breadth for finding frame size.

Section 5: Body Mass Index—Further reviews the use of BMI in evaluating body weight and provides reference ranges for dialysis and transplant patients. Formulas for adjusting BMI for amputation are presented.

Section 6: Skinfold Measurements—Provides instructions for performing skinfold measurements and calculating arm fat and arm muscle areas.

Section 7: Subjective Global Assessment—Lists and describes the components involved in performing Subjective Global Assessment.

Section 8: Laboratory Values in Dialysis Patients—Covers factors that can affect the interpretation of laboratory values, particularly in relation to dialysis patients. Includes discussion of specific issues regarding albumin, calcium, and parathyroid hormone tests.

Section 9: Energy Estimation—Describes two methods for determining energy needs in CKD patients.

Section 10: Intradialytic Parenteral Nutrition (IDPN)—Reviews the use of IDPN in dialysis patients. Provides guidelines for determining the components of IDPN and for monitoring laboratory data and nutritional status in the patient receiving IDPN.

Section 11: Vitamins and Minerals in Chronic Kidney Disease—Offers a detailed review of the vitamin and mineral status of CKD patients. Discusses potential toxicities and the results of inadequate levels of specific nutrients. Provides recommendations for supplementation of vitamins.

Section 12: Physical Signs of Nutrient Deficiencies/Excesses—Presents a guide for evaluating physical symptoms suggestive of nutrient-specific deficiencies/excesses by body area. Lists the nutrients to consider when these physical symptoms are present.

Section 13: Reasons for Inadequate Response to Erythropoietin (EPO)—Lists the conditions that may contribute to hyporesponsiveness to EPO therapy.

Section 14: Glomerular Filtration Rate and Creatinine Clearance—Provides formulas for determining glomerular filtration rate from serum creatinine and from creatinine clearance.

Section 15: Protein Catabolic Rate (PCR) and Protein Equivalent of Nitrogen Appearance Rate (PNA)—Describes the difference between PCR and PNA. Formulas are provided for calculating PCR, PNA, and the normalized PNA (nPNA).

Section 16: Dialysis Adequacy—Explains the use and determination of dialysis adequacy in hemodialysis and peritoneal dialysis patients. Provides formulas for determining urea reduction ratio (URR) and Kt/V, and describes the incorporation of residual renal function into Kt/V for hemodialysis patients. Recommended targets for adequacy levels from the National Kidney Foundation's Kidney Disease Outcomes Quality Initiative (K/DOQI) Guidelines are included.

Section 17: Volume and Body Surface Area Calculations—Presents formulas for determining total body water volume and body surface area in dialysis patients. Also includes guidelines for adjusting volume and body surface area for amputation.

Section 18: Cardiovascular Disease—Reviews the latest available information regarding cardiovascular disease in CKD patients. Discusses hypertension, hyperlipidemia, hyperglycemia, tobacco use, physical inactivity, homocysteine, and cardiovascular calcification. Recommendations from a variety of agencies for the prevention and treatment of cardiovascular disease are presented.

Section 19: Exercise and Rehabilitation—Describes the five core areas identified as fundamental in the rehabilitation of CKD patients, with emphasis on exercise and its relation to nutritional status.

Section 20: Immunosuppressant Drugs and Nutritional Side Effects—Lists the major immunosuppressant drugs currently in use and the possible nutritional side effects from the drugs. Also presents recommendations for nutrition intervention for the side effects.

This publication is intended to provide the practitioner with the latest information and recommendations regarding nutritional assessment and care of CKD patients and to supply the tools necessary to adequately assess nutritional status in patients with CKD. Each section has been thoroughly researched, and the most recent scientific literature and expert opinion used to compose the material presented. The guide is written to complement the nutrition assessment sections presented in the *Guidelines for Nutrition Care of Renal Patients,* 3rd edition, but it can also be used on its own as a reference manual for those who provide care to the renal population.

Abbreviations

AFA	mid-upper arm fat area
AHA	American Heart Association
AI	Adequate Intakes
AMA	arm muscle area
ATP III	Adult Treatment Panel III
BCG	bromcresol green
BCP	bromcresol purple
BEE	basal energy expenditure
BEI	bioelectric impedence
BMI	body mass index
BSA	body surface area
BUN	blood urea nitrogen
BW	body weight
Ca x P	calcium-phosphorus product
CANUSA	Canada-USA Peritoneal Dialysis Study
CAPD	continuous ambulatory peritoneal dialysis
CAVH	continuous arteriovenous hemodialysis
CCPD	continuous cyclic peritoneal dialysis
Ccr	creatinine clearance
CHD	coronary heart disease
CKD	chronic kidney disease
Cr	creatinine
Cu	urea clearance
CVD	cardiovascular disease
DFO	deferoxamine
DOPPS	Dialysis Outcomes and Practice Patterns Study
DRI	Dietary Reference Intakes
DUN	dialysate urea nitrogen
ECF	extracellular fluid
EPO	erythropoietin
ESRD	end-stage renal disease
FDA	Federal Drug Administration
FFM	fat free mass
GFR	glomerular filtration rate
GI	gastrointestinal
GPX	glutathione peroxidase
GTF	glucose tolerance factor
HDL	high density lipoprotein
HEMO	Hemodialysis Study
HgbA1C	hemoglobin A1C (glycosylated hemoglobin)
HIV	human immunodeficiency virus
ht	height

IBW	ideal body weight
IDPN	intradialytic parenteral nutrition
IF	intrinsic factor
i-PTH	intact parathyroid hormone
IV	intravenous
JNC VI	Sixth Joint National Committee on the Prevention, Detection, Evaluation, and Treatment of High Blood Pressure
kcal	kilocalories
K/DOQI	Kidney Disease Outcomes Quality Initiative
Kru	residual renal clearance of urea
Kt/V	measure of dose of dialysis
LDL	low density lipoprotein
LORAC	Life Options Rehabilitation Advisory Council
MAC	mid-upper arm circumference
MDRD	Modification of Diet in Renal Disease
NHANES	National Health and Nutrition Evaluation Survey
NCEP	National Cholesterol Education Program
NHLBI	National Heart, Lung, and Blood Institute
NIH	National Institutes of Health
NIPD	nightly intermittent peritoneal dialysis
NKF	National Kidney Foundation
nPCR	normalized protein catabolic rate
nPNA	normalized protein equivalent of nitrogen appearance
PCR	protein catabolic rate
PLP	pyridoxal-5'-phosphate
PNA	protein equivalent of nitrogen appearance
PTH	parathyroid hormone
RDA	Recommended Dietary Allowances
REE	resting energy expenditure
SBW	standard body weight
SGA	subjective global assessment
TLC	therapeutic lifestyle changes
TPN	total parenteral nutrition
TSF	triceps skinfold
UA	urea appearance
UF	ultrafiltration volume
UNA	urea nitrogen appearance
URR	urea reduction ratio
UUN	urinary urea nitrogen
V	volume
wt	weight

Section 1
Federal Regulations

Minimum requirements for adequate provision of patient care in outpatient dialysis units are set by the federal government. Professional organizations must adhere to these minimums. These regulations can be found in the Code of Federal Regulations, Title 42, Volume 2, Part 405, Subpart U—Conditions for Coverage of Suppliers of End-Stage Renal Disease (ESRD).

Regulations

405.2102 Definitions: Qualified Personnel

(b) *Dietitian.* A person who: (1) is eligible for registration by The American Dietetic Association under its requirements in effect on the publication of these regulations (June 3, 1976), and has at least 1 year of experience in clinical nutrition; or (2) has a baccalaureate or advanced degree with major studies in food and nutrition or dietetics, and has at least 1 year of experience in clinical nutrition.

405.2137 Condition: Patient long-term program and patient care plan

Each facility maintains for each patient a written long-term program and a written patient care plan to ensure that each patient receives the appropriate modality of care and the appropriate care within that modality. The patient, or where appropriate, parent or legal guardian, is involved with the health team in the planning of care. A copy of the current program and plan accompany the patient on interfacility transfer.

(a) *Standard: Patient long-term program.* There is a written long-term program representing the selection of a suitable treatment modality (ie, dialysis or transplantation) and dialysis setting (eg, home, self-care) for each patient.

   (1) The program is developed by a professional team which includes but is not limited to the physician director of the dialysis facility or center where the patient is currently being treated, a physician director of a center or facility which offers self-care dialysis training (if not available at the location where the patient is being treated), a transplant surgeon, a qualified nurse responsible for nursing services, a qualified dietitian, and a qualified social worker.

   (2) The program is formally reviewed and revised in writing as necessary by a team which includes but is not limited to the physician director of the dialysis facility or center where the patient is presently being treated, in addition to the other personnel listed in paragraph (a) (1) of this section at least every 12 months or more often as indicated by the patient's response to treatment. [See Sec. 405.2161(b)(1) and Sec. 405.2170(a).*]

   (3) The patient, parent, or legal guardian, as appropriate, is involved in the development of the patient's long-term program, and due consideration is given to his preferences.

---

*Cited sections are omitted from this book.

(4) A copy of the patient's long-term program accompanies the patient on interfacility transfer or is sent within 1 working day.

(b) *Standard: Patient care plan.* There is a written patient care plan for each patient of an ESRD facility [including home dialysis patients under the supervision of the ESRD facility; see Sec.405.2163(e)], based on the nature of the patient's illness, the treatment prescribed, and an assessment of the patient's needs.

(1) The patient care plan is personalized for the individual, reflects the psychological, social, and functional needs of the patient, and indicates the ESRD and other care required as well as the individualized modifications in approach necessary to achieve long-term and short-term goals.

(2) The plan is developed by a professional team consisting of at least the physician responsible for the patient's ESRD care, a qualified nurse responsible for nursing services, a qualified social worker, and a qualified dietitian.

(3) The patient, parent, or legal guardian, as appropriate, is involved in the development of the care plan, and due consideration is given to his or her preferences.

(4) The care plan for patients whose medical condition has not become stabilized is reviewed at least monthly by the professional patient care team described in paragraph (b) (2) of this section. For patients whose condition has become stabilized, the care plan is reviewed every 6 months. The care plan is revised as necessary to ensure that it provides for patient's ongoing needs.

(5) If the patient is transferred to another facility, the care plan is sent with the patient or within 1 working day.

(6) For a home dialysis patient whose care is under the supervision of the ESRD facility, the care plan provides for periodic monitoring of the patient's home adaptation, including provisions for visits to the home by qualified facility personnel to the extent appropriate. [See 405.2163(e)].

(7) Beginning July 1, 1991, for a home dialysis patient, and beginning January 1, 1994, for any dialysis patient, who uses erythropoietin (EPO) in the home, the plan must provide for monitoring home use of EPO that includes the following:

(i) Review of the diet and fluid intake for indiscretions as indicated by hyperkalemia and elevated blood pressure secondary to volume overload.

(ii) Review of medications to ensure adequate provision of supplemental iron.

(iii) Ongoing evaluations of hematocrit and iron stores.

(iv) A reevaluation of the dialysis prescription taking into account the patient's increased appetite and red blood cell volume.

(v) A method for physician follow-up on blood tests and a mechanism (such as a patient log) for keeping the physician informed of the results.

(vi) Training of the patient to identify the signs and symptoms of hypotension and hypertension.

(vii) The decrease or discontinuance of EPO if hypertension is uncontrollable.

405.2163 Condition: Minimal service requirements for a renal dialysis facility or renal dialysis center

The facility must provide dialysis services, as well as adequate laboratory, social, and dietetic services to meet the needs of the ESRD patient.

(d) *Standard: Dietetic services.* Each patient is evaluated as to his nutritional needs by the attending physician and by a qualified dietitian [Sec. 405.2102] who has an employment or contractual relationship with the facility. The dietitian, in consultation with the attending physician, is responsible for assessing the nutritional and dietetic needs of each patient, recommending therapeutic diets, counseling patients and their families on prescribed diets, and monitoring adherence and response to diets.

(e) *Standard: Self-dialysis support services.* The renal dialysis facility or center furnishing self-dialysis training upon completion of the patient's training, furnishes (either directly, under agreement or by arrangement with another ESRD facility) the following services:

(1) Surveillance of the patient's home adaptation, including provisions for visits to the home or the facility;

(2) Consultation for the patient with a qualified social worker and a qualified dietitian;

(3) A recordkeeping system which assures continuity of care;

(4) Installation and maintenance of equipment;

(5) Testing and appropriate treatment of the water; and

(6) Ordering of supplies on an ongoing basis.

405.2171 Condition: Minimal service requirements for a renal transplantation center

(c) *Standard: Dietetic services.* Each patient is evaluated as to his nutritional needs by the attending physician and by a qualified dietitian [Sec. 405.2102] who has an employment or contractual relationship with the facility. The dietitian, in consultation with the attending physician, is responsible for assessing the nutritional and dietetic needs of each patient, recommending therapeutic diets, counseling patients and their families on prescribed diets, and monitoring adherence and response to diets.

Section 2
Height Determination

An accurate height is best obtained by direct measurement rather than from the self-report of the patient. Height is frequently overreported, especially in those older than 60 years of age, with men overestimating height more than women (1–4). In dialysis patients, self-reported height has been shown to overestimate actual height (5). The self-reported height of dialysis patients may be overestimated to an even greater extent than in other populations, possibly due to the high incidence of renal bone disease (5).

Direct Measurement

Height in adults is measured in the standing position using a stadiometer. A stadiometer consists of a nonstretch tape or measuring stick attached to a vertical surface, such as a wall or a rigid free-standing measuring device, and a movable block, attached to the vertical surface at a right angle, that can be brought down to the crown of the head (6–8). If measuring against a wall, there should be no baseboard and the floor should not be carpeted (7). An anthropometer, a vertical graduated rod with a moveable horizontal rod, can also be used to measure height (7). When measuring height, the patient should stand erect with feet together and weight distributed equally on both feet (6,7). When possible, the heels, buttocks, shoulder blades, and head should touch the wall or the vertical surface of the measuring device (6-8). Arms should hang freely at the sides with palms facing the thighs (6–8). The patient is asked to look straight ahead, take a deep breath, and stand tall to aid the straightening of the spine (7,8). The movable block is brought down until it touches the crown of the head (6,8). Measurement is taken at maximum inspiration with the examiner's eyes level with the headboard (7,8). Measurement is recorded to the nearest 0.1 cm (6,7).

Indirect Measurement

For patients who are unable to stand for height measurement, two methods are available for estimating height.

Estimating Height—Method 1: Arm Span

In both men and women the arm span measurement is roughly equal to height (within 10%) and does not change significantly with age (7,9). For elderly patients, arm span estimates stature at maturity before age-related bone loss (7). Arm span can be difficult to measure in patients who are unable to stretch out their arms adequately, and chest measurements can be altered by lung disease, kyphosis, or osteoporosis (7).

Arm span is measured with the arms fully extended at shoulder level and perpendicular to the patient's body, palms facing forward (7,9). Measurement is taken across the back from the tip of one middle finger to the tip of the other middle finger (7,9). For bedridden patients, measurement is taken between the tips of the middle fingers with the measuring tape passing over the clavicles (10).

Estimating Height—Method 2: Knee Height

Measurement of knee height is highly correlated with stature and decreases little with age (7–9). Knee height is best measured using knee calipers while the patient lies in a supine position with the knee and ankle flexed to 90 degrees (8,10). If it is not possible to take the measurement with the patient lying down, it is acceptable to measure knee height with the patient in the seated position, with one leg crossed over the opposite knee (9). Measurement is preferably taken on the outside of the left leg or the non-access leg if the patient has a leg access (8,10).

The fixed blade of the calipers is placed under the heel with the other blade on the anterior surface of the thigh just proximal to the patella (8,10). The shaft of the calipers is held parallel to the shaft of the tibia, and pressure is applied to compress the tissue (8,10). Two successive measurements should be taken and recorded to the nearest 0.1 cm (10). The mean of the two measurements is used in the following formulas to estimate stature (11):

Stature (women) = (1.83 × knee height) – (0.24 × age) + 84.88

Stature (men) = (2.02 × knee height) – (0.04 × age) + 64.19

Where knee height is measured in cm.

References

1. Spencer EA, Appleby PN, Davey GK, Key TJ. Validity of self-reported height and weight in 4,808 EPIC-Oxford participants. *Public Health Nutr.* 2002;5:561–565.

2. DelPrete LR, Caldwell M, English C, Banspach SW, Lefebvre C. Self-reported and measured weights and heights of participants in community-based weight-loss programs. *J Am Diet Assoc.* 1992;92:1483–1486.

3. Palta M, Prineas RJ, Berman R, Hannan P. Comparison of self-reported and measured height and weight. *Am J Epidemiol.* 1982;115:223–230.

4. Kuczmarski MF, Kuczmarski RJ, Najjar M. Effects of age on validity of self-reported height, weight, and body mass index: findings from the Third National Health and Nutrition Examination Survey, 1988–1994. *J Am Diet Assoc.* 2001;101:28–34.

5. Schneider RD, Wilkens K. Actual and self-reported height in patients with end-stage renal disease. *J Ren Nutr.* 1997;7:83–89.

6. Frisancho AR. *Anthropometric Standards for the Assessment of Growth and Nutritional Status.* Ann Arbor, Mich: University of Michigan Press; 1990.

7. Grant A, DeHoog S. *Nutritional Assessment and Support.* 5th ed. Seattle, Wash: Grant and DeHoog Publishers; 1999.

8. Gibson RS. *Principles of Nutritional Assessment.* New York, NY: Oxford University Press; 1990.

9. Callahan C, ed. Ask CRN. *J Ren Nutr.* 1996;6:51.

10. Matarese LE, Gottschlich MM. *Contemporary Nutrition Support Practice: A Clinical Guide.* Philadelphia, Pa: WB Saunders; 1998.

11. Chumlea WC. Methods of nutritional anthropometric assessment for special groups. In: Lohman TG, Roche AG, Martorell R, eds. *Anthropometric Standardization Reference Manual.* Champaign, Ill: Human Kinectics; 1988:93–95.

Section 3
Evaluation of Body Weight

Ideal Body Weight

The term *ideal body weight* (IBW) has historically been used to define the weight associated with the lowest mortality for normal individuals of a given height, age range, sex, and frame size. *Desirable body weight* and *healthy weight* are other terms frequently used to express the same concept.

The Metropolitan Height and Weight Tables have generally been the most widely used for determination of IBW. These tables provide the weights associated with the lowest mortality rate by frame size and are based on mortality data collected during 20-year periods from healthy subjects who purchased life insurance policies (1). There has been some concern regarding the use of these tables, however. The tables have been criticized because the populations on which they are based underrepresent the lower socioeconomic class, women, minorities, and the elderly, and thus do not accurately represent the US population (2–6). Also criticized is the arbitrary definition of frame size (2,6). For the 1983 table, frame size was determined by the elbow breadth definition derived from the first National Health and Nutrition Evaluation Survey (NHANES I) population, but the weights associated with the frame size were from the Metropolitan Insurance policyholder population (6). The 1983 table, which is the most current table available, can be readily found on the Internet or may be obtained by contacting MetLife (1 Madison Ave, New York, NY 10010-3690, info@metlife.com). Methods for determining frame size are presented in Section 4.

The use of *body mass index* (BMI) for evaluation of body weight has been emphasized recently. Recommendations for a healthy weight (or IBW) have been based on the BMI range that yields the lowest morbidity and mortality rates. Using the BMI level associated with the lowest morbidity and mortality, IBW can be calculated. Section 5 provides the BMI levels associated with lowest morbidity and mortality for the general US population. For individuals with renal failure, recommended BMI levels are also provided in Section 5, and these levels can be used in the formula to calculate IBW:

Formula 1: IBW (kg) = BMI × ht^2

Where:

BMI = Recommended BMI or BMI associated with the lowest mortality
ht = height (m)

BMI has been universally adopted as the standard for defining obesity. The World Health Organization, National Institutes of Health, and the American Health Foundation's Expert Panel on Healthy Weight recommend using BMI to evaluate body weight (7–9). BMI correlates both with overall mortality and with morbidity due to diabetes, cerebrovascular disease, and cardiovascular disease and is the favored measure in epidemiological studies to evaluate relative risk of disease due to excess weight (2,8). Because of the simplicity of calculating BMI, it can be applied easily in the clinical setting (8,10). Frame size measurements are not necessary and tables are not required to determine BMI or to calculate IBW from BMI (2,10). Table 3.1 provides the weights corresponding to BMI levels considered appropriate for dialysis patients.

Table 3.1   Weights Corresponding to BMI Levels of 23 to 25 by Height

Height		Weight	
in	cm	lb	kg
58	147	109–119	49.7–54.0
59	150	114–124	51.8–56.3
60	152	117–127	53.1–57.8
61	155	122–132	55.3–60.1
62	157	125–136	56.7–61.6
63	160	130–141	58.9–64.0
64	163	134–146	61.1–66.4
65	165	138–150	62.6–68.1
66	168	143–155	64.9–70.6
67	170	146–159	66.5–72.3
68	173	151–165	68.8–74.8
69	175	155–168	70.4–76.6
70	178	160–174	72.9–79.2
71	180	164–178	74.5–81.0
72	183	169–184	77.0–83.7
73	185	173–188	78.7–85.6
74	188	179–194	81.3–88.4
75	191	184–200	83.5–90.7
76	193	189–205	85.7–93.2
77	196	194–210	88.0–95.6

Standard Body Weight

An alternative to IBW is *standard body weight* (SBW). SBW is the median body weight (50th percentile) of healthy normal Americans of the same height, age range, sex, and frame size (5,11). The SBW values are typically obtained from the National Health and Nutrition Evaluation Surveys (NHANES) conducted by the National Center for Health Statistics (12). Three NHANES studies have been completed to date (NHANES I from 1971 to 1975, NHANES II from 1976 to 1980, and NHANES III from 1988 to 1994), and as of 1999, NHANES has become a continuous survey without breaks between cycles (13,14). For the NHANES data, skeletal frame size is determined using elbow breadth. The method for determining frame size by elbow breadth is presented in Section 4.

The use of the NHANES data for body weight evaluation has been recommended instead of the Metropolitan Life Insurance data by some (3,5,12). The NHANES data is gathered from large numbers of noninstitutionalized males and females (age range, 1 to 74 years) from the US population and is considered a more representative sample of that population than the Metropolitan Life Insurance data (3,5,6). Older individuals were included in the NHANES studies but not in the Metropolitan Life Insurance studies, which limited participant age to 59 years or younger (5,6).

One disadvantage of using the SBW and the NHANES data is the definition of SBW as the *median* weight of the NHANES population. The NHANES studies have shown that the body weight for height of the average American increased between the NHANES II study and the NHANES III study, with the prevalence of obesity (defined as BMI ≥ 30) also increasing (14,15). Data for NHANES 1999–2000 show further increases in the prevalence of obesity for men and women in all age groups and for all racial/ethnic groups studied (14). As the weight of Americans increases, the SBW for a given individual will also increase. This was one reason for rejecting the use of population norms by the American Health Foundation's Expert Panel on Healthy Weight (16). Additionally, SBW is not based on mortality or morbidity data, so it is unknown if the SBW is the weight that achieves lowest mortality or morbidity. Finally, frame size in the NHANES studies was determined using elbow breadth, which requires the use of a particular measuring device and may not be feasible for many clinicians (10).

NHANES tables are provided in this section (Tables 3.2 through 3.8). Tables 3.2 through 3.7 present the percentiles of weight by height and frame size derived from the combined NHANES I and II data sets. Table 3.8 presents the percentiles of weight by age derived from the NHANES III data set. At this time, the frame size categorization of weight by height is not available for NHANES III data.

Table 3.2   Selected Percentiles of Weight by Height for US Men and Women with Small Frames, 25 to 54 years old— NHANES I and II Data

Height		Wt (kg)							Height		Wt (kg)						
in	cm	5	10	15	50	85	90	95	in	cm	5	10	15	50	85	90	95
				Men									Women				
62	157	46*	50*	52*	64	71*	74*	77*	58	147	37*	43	43	52	58	62	66*
63	160	48*	51*	53	61	70	75*	79*	59	150	42	43	44	53	63	69	72
64	163	49*	53	55	66	76	76	80*	60	152	42	44	45	53	63	65	70
65	165	52	53	58	66	77	81	84	61	155	44	46	47	54	64	66	72
66	168	56	57	59	67	78	83	84	62	157	44	47	48	55	63	64	70
67	170	56	60	62	71	82	83	88	63	160	46	48	49	55	65	68	79
68	173	56	59	62	71	79	82	85	64	163	49	50	51	57	67	68	74
69	175	57*	62	65	74	84	87	88*	65	165	50	52	53	60	70	72	80
70	178	59*	62*	67	75	87	86*	90*	66	168	46*	49*	54	58	65	71*	74*
71	180	60*	64*	70	76	79	88*	91*	67	170	47*	50*	52*	59	70*	72*	76*
72	183	62*	65*	67*	74	87*	89*	93*	68	173	48*	51*	53*	62	71*	73*	77*
73	185	63*	67*	69*	79*	89*	91*	94*	69	175	49*	52*	54*	63*	72*	74*	78*
74	188	65*	68*	71*	80*	90*	92*	96*	70	178	50*	53*	55*	64*	73*	75*	79*

*Value estimated through linear regression equation.

Adapted from and reproduced with permission by the *American Journal of Clinical Nutrition*. © Am J Clin Nutr. American Society for Clinical Nutrition (6).

Table 3.3   Selected Percentiles of Weight by Height for US Men and Women with Medium Frames, 25 to 54 years old—NHANES I and II Data

Height		Wt (kg)							Height		Wt (kg)						
in	cm	5	10	15	50	85	90	95	in	cm	5	10	15	50	85	90	95
					Men									Women			
62	157	51*	55*	58*	68	81*	83*	87*	58	147	41*	46*	50	63	77	75*	79*
63	160	52*	56*	59*	71	82*	85*	89*	59	150	47	50	52	66	76	79	85
64	163	54*	60	61	71	83	84	90*	60	152	47	50	52	60	77	79	85
65	165	59	62	65	74	87	90	94	61	155	47	49	51	61	73	78	86
66	168	58	61	65	75	85	87	93	62	157	49	50	52	61	73	77	83
67	170	62	66	68	77	89	93	100	63	160	49	51	53	62	77	80	88
68	173	60	64	66	78	89	92	97	64	163	50	52	54	62	76	82	87
69	175	63	66	68	78	90	93	97	65	165	52	54	55	63	75	80	89
70	178	64	66	70	81	90	93	97	66	168	52	54	55	63	75	78	83
71	180	62	68	70	81	92	96	100	67	170	54	56	57	65	79	82	88
72	183	68	71	74	84	97	100	104	68	173	58	59	60	67	77	85	87
73	185	70	72	75	85	100	101	104	69	175	49*	58	60	68	79	82	87*
74	188	68*	76	77	88	100	100	104*	70	178	50*	54*	57*	70	80*	83*	87*

*Value estimated through linear regression equation.
Adapted from and reproduced with permission by the *American Journal of Clinical Nutrition.* © Am J Clin Nutr. American Society for Clinical Nutrition (6).

Table 3.4   Selected Percentiles of Weight by Height for US Men and Women with Large Frames, 25 to 54 years old—NHANES I and II data

Height		Wt (kg)							Height		Wt (kg)						
in	cm	5	10	15	50	85	90	95	in	cm	5	10	15	50	85	90	95
					Men									Women			
62	157	57*	62*	66*	82*	99*	103*	108*	58	147	56*	63*	67*	86*	105*	110*	117*
63	160	58*	63*	67*	83*	100*	104*	109*	59	150	56*	62*	67*	78	105*	109*	116*
64	163	59*	64*	68*	84*	101*	105*	110*	60	152	55*	62*	66*	87	104*	109*	116*
65	165	60*	65*	69*	79	102*	106*	111*	61	155	54*	64	66	81	105	117	115*
66	168	60*	65*	75	84	103	106*	112*	62	157	59	61	65	81	103	107	113
67	170	62*	70	71	84	102	111	113*	63	160	58	63	67	83	105	109	119
68	173	63*	74	76	86	101	104	114*	64	163	59	62	63	79	102	104	112
69	175	68	71	74	89	103	105	114	65	165	59	61	63	81	103	109	114
70	178	68	72	74	87	106	112	114	66	168	55	58	62	75	95	100	107
71	180	73	78	82	91	113	116	123	67	170	58	60	65	80	100	108	114
72	183	73	76	78	91	109	112	121	68	173	51*	66	66	76	104	105	111*
73	185	72	77	79	93	106	107	116	69	175	50*	57*	68	79	105	104*	111*
74	188	69*	74*	82	92	105	115*	120*	70	178	50*	56*	61*	76	99*	104*	110*

*Value estimated through linear regression equation.
Adapted from and reproduced with permission by the *American Journal of Clinical Nutrition.* © Am J Clin Nutr. American Society for Clinical Nutrition (6).

Table 3.5 Selected Percentiles of Weight by Height for US Men and Women with Small Frames, 55 to 74 years old—NHANES I and II Data

Height		Wt (kg)							Height		Wt (kg)						
in	cm	5	10	15	50	85	90	95	in	cm	5	10	15	50	85	90	95
				Men									Women				
62	157	45*	49*	56	61	68	73*	77*	58	147	39*	46	48	54	63	65	71*
63	160	47*	49	51	62	71	71	79*	59	150	41	45	48	55	66	68	74
64	163	47	50	54	63	72	74	80	60	152	43	45	47	54	67	70	73
65	165	48	54	59	70	80	90	90	61	155	43	43	45	56	65	70	71
66	168	51	55	59	68	77	80	84	62	157	47	49	52	58	67	69	73
67	170	55	60	61	69	79	81	88	63	160	42*	45	49	58	67	68	74*
68	173	54*	54	58	70	79	81	86*	64	163	43*	47	49	60	68	70	75*
69	175	56*	59*	63	75	81	84*	88*	65	165	43*	47*	49*	60	69*	72*	75*
70	178	57*	61*	63*	76	83*	86*	89*	66	168	44*	48*	50*	68	70*	72*	76*
71	180	59*	62*	65*	69	85*	87*	91*	67	170	45*	48*	51*	61*	71*	73*	77*
72	183	60*	64*	66*	76*	86*	89*	92*	68	173	45*	49*	51*	61*	71*	74*	77*
73	185	62*	65*	68*	78*	88*	90*	94*	69	175	46*	49*	52*	62*	72*	74*	78*
74	188	63*	67*	69*	77*	89*	92*	95*	70	178	47*	50*	52*	63*	73*	75*	79*

*Value estimated through linear regression equation.
Adapted from and reproduced with permission by the *American Journal of Clinical Nutrition*. © Am J Clin Nutr. American Society for Clinical Nutrition (6).

Table 3.6 Selected Percentiles of Weight by Height for US Men and Women with Medium Frames, 55 to 74 years old—NHANES I and II Data

Height		Wt (kg)							Height		Wt (kg)						
in	cm	5	10	15	50	85	90	95	in	cm	5	10	15	50	85	90	95
				Men									Women				
62	157	50*	54*	59	68	77	81*	85*	58	147	40	44	49	57	72	82	85
63	160	51*	57	60	70	80	82	87*	59	150	47	49	52	62	74	78	86
64	163	55	59	62	71	82	83	91	60	152	47	50	52	65	76	79	86
65	165	56	60	64	72	83	86	89	61	155	49	51	54	64	78	81	86
66	168	57	62	66	74	83	84	89	62	157	49	53	54	64	78	82	88
67	170	59	64	66	78	87	89	94	63	160	52	54	55	65	79	83	89
68	173	62	66	68	78	89	95	101	64	163	51	54	57	66	78	81	87
69	175	62	66	68	77	90	93	99	65	165	54	56	59	67	78	84	88
70	178	62	68	71	80	90	95	101	66	168	54	57	57	66	79	85	88
71	180	68	70	72	84	94	97	101	67	170	51*	59	61	72	82	85	89*
72	183	66*	65	69	81	96	97	101*	68	173	52*	56*	59*	70	83*	86*	90*
73	185	68*	72*	79	88	93	99*	103*	69	175	53*	57*	60*	72*	84*	87*	91*
74	188	69*	73*	76*	95	98*	101*	104*	70	178	54*	58*	61*	73*	85*	88*	92*

*Value estimated through linear regression equation.
Adapted from and reproduced with permission by the *American Journal of Clinical Nutrition*. © Am J Clin Nutr. American Society for Clinical Nutrition (6).

Table 3.7   Selected Percentiles of Weight by Height for US Men and Women with Large Frames, 55 to 74 years old—NHANES I and II Data

Height		Wt (kg)							Height		Wt (kg)						
in	cm	5	10	15	50	85	90	95	in	cm	5	10	15	50	85	90	95
				Men									**Women**				
62	157	54*	59*	63*	77*	91*	95*	100*	58	147	53*	59*	63*	92	95*	99*	104*
63	160	55*	60*	64*	80	92*	96*	101*	59	150	54*	59*	63*	78	95*	99*	105*
64	163	57*	62*	65*	77	94*	97*	102*	60	152	54*	65	69	78	87	88	105*
65	165	58*	63*	73	79	89	98*	103*	61	155	64	68	69	79	94	95	106
66	168	59*	67	73	80	101	102	105*	62	157	59	61	63	82	93	101	111
67	170	65	71	73	85	103	108	112	63	160	61	65	67	80	100	102	118
68	173	67	71	73	83	95	98	111	64	163	60	65	67	77	97	102	119
69	175	65	70	74	84	96	98	105	65	165	60	66	69	80	98	102	111
70	178	68	73	77	87	102	104	117	66	168	57*	60	63	82	98	105	109*
71	180	65*	70	70	84	102	109	111*	67	170	58*	64*	68	80	105	104*	109*
72	183	67*	76	81	90	108	112	112*	68	173	58*	64*	68*	79	100*	104*	110*
73	185	68*	73*	76*	88	105*	108*	113*	69	175	59*	65*	69*	85*	101*	105*	110*
74	188	69*	74*	78*	89	106*	109*	114*	70	178	60*	65*	69*	85*	101*	105*	111*

*Value estimated through linear regression equation.
Adapted from and reproduced with permission by the *American Journal of Clinical Nutrition*. © Am J Clin Nutr. American Society for Clinical Nutrition (6).

Table 3.8   Selected Percentiles of Weight by Age for US Men and Women, 20 Years and Older, 1988–1994—NHANES III Data

Age (years)	Wt (kg)								
	5	10	15	25	50	75	85	90	95
					Men				
20–29	57.7	60.9	63.0	67.0	75.0	85.3	93.3	99.0	107.6
30–39	61.9	64.6	67.3	71.9	80.0	91.3	98.8	102.9	112.7
40–49	61.5	66.0	68.6	74.4	82.1	93.9	101.5	105.7	116.5
50–59	63.5	68.2	72.0	75.8	84.0	94.0	100.7	105.2	114.2
60–69	61.1	64.5	67.6	72.8	82.3	92.4	98.4	102.0	107.4
70–79	58.5	62.0	64.2	68.8	77.9	86.9	93.5	96.1	103.2
80 and over	52.0	56.1	58.4	63.7	70.8	78.7	84.2	87.9	93.0
					Women				
20–29	46.8	49.1	50.5	53.8	60.5	71.5	79.6	85.9	98.4
30–39	48.3	51.1	53.4	57.0	65.5	78.5	89.0	96.3	105.9
40–49	49.6	53.1	55.7	59.1	68.5	79.8	88.1	95.2	104.7
50–59	51.8	54.6	57.1	61.4	71.5	84.5	91.6	97.0	109.0
60–69	49.5	52.5	55.4	59.2	68.8	79.4	86.9	91.9	100.3
70–79	45.7	50.2	52.9	56.8	64.7	75.8	82.1	86.1	97.2
80 and over	41.8	45.5	47.9	51.9	59.7	67.9	72.3	76.7	84.7

Adapted from National Center for Health Statistics Data Tables: Weight in pounds for males 20 years and over, number of examined persons, standard error of the mean, and selected percentiles, by race-ethnicity, age: United States, 1988–1994. Available at: http://www.cdc.gov/nchs/about/major/nhanes/wgtmal.pdf. Accessed November 8, 2002 (17); and National Center for Health Statistics Data Tables: Weight in pounds for females 20 years and over, number of examined persons, standard error of the mean, and selected percentiles, by race-ethnicity, age: United States, 1988–1994. Available at: http://www.cdc.gov/nchs/about/major/nhanes/wgtfem.pdf. Accessed November 8, 2002 (18).

Evaluating Body Weight in Renal Disease

There is no current standard for which method to use in evaluating body weight for individuals with chronic kidney disease (CKD). The National Kidney Foundation (NKF) Kidney Disease Outcome Quality Initiative (K/DOQI) Clinical Practice Guidelines for Nutrition in Chronic Renal Failure recommend using SBW and NHANES II data to evaluate body weight in dialysis patients. These guidelines suggest that the target body weight be between 90% and 110% of SBW (12). The K/DOQI Nutrition Guidelines and the K/DOQI Clinical Practice Guidelines for Chronic Kidney Disease also recommend using BMI to evaluate weight in dialysis patients (10,12). They suggest that dry weight be maintained in the upper 50th percentile for dialysis patients, which corresponds to a BMI of no less than approximately 23.6 for men and 24.3 for women (10,12,19). It is left to the practitioner to determine which method to use for evaluating body weight.

Adjusting Body Weight for Amputation

Weight of an amputated limb must be considered when determining IBW/SBW. The IBW/SBW provided directly by the tables or calculated using BMI will overestimate the actual IBW/SBW of the individual with the amputation. The following method can be used to adjust IBW/SBW for the amputated limb:

1. Determine the percentage of total body weight contributed by the missing limb. (Section 17 provides a table of the percentage of total body weight contributed by certain segments of the body.)
2. Find the IBW or SBW for the individual's height using one of the methods listed earlier in this section.
3. Multiply this weight by [100 – (% weight of amputation)] and divide the result by 100.

Example: For a 5 ft 10 in (178 cm) male weighing 163 lb (74 kg) with a leg amputated to the knee:

1. The percentage of total body weight contributed by the missing limb = 1.5 (foot) + 4.4 (calf) = 5.9%
2. IBW (using BMI method and a BMI level of 24) = $24 \times (1.78)^2 = 76.0$ kg
3. Adjusted IBW = $\dfrac{76.0 \times [100 - (5.9)]}{100} = \dfrac{76.0 \times (94.1)}{100} = 71.5$ kg

Adjustment for Obesity

In obesity, it has been common practice to adjust body weight in reference to IBW or SBW for the purposes of determining energy needs. The rationale behind this method is that an obese person has a greater percentage of body fat, which is much less metabolically active and requires less energy than fat-free mass (FFM) (1,2). Using the obese individual's actual body weight to determine needs would lead to an overestimation of energy. However, an increase in weight consists of an increase in not only fat tissue but also in FFM (2–4). Thus, using IBW or SBW for an obese individual would underestimate energy needs. It has been found that FFM correlates closely with resting energy expenditure (REE) in normal-weight and obese subjects, (5–10) and thus the common practice has been to consider the increase in FFM that accompanies accrual of fat tissue and adjust body weight accordingly. Various studies have looked at the percentage of FFM in obese tissue, and estimates range from 22% to 33% FFM for women and 19% to 38% FFM for men. To adjust body weight using this rationale, Formula 2 can be used (for individuals > 120% IBW) (2–4,10).

Formula 2: Adjusted Weight (kg or lb) = [(BW – IBW) × FFM factor] +IBW

Where:

BW = actual body weight
IBW = ideal body weight or standard body weight
FFM factor = 0.22–0.33 Women
　　　　　　0.19–0.38 Men

Another formula for determining adjusted body weight has been proposed by the NKF-K/DOQI Clinical Practice Guidelines for Nutrition in Chronic Renal Failure for use with individuals weighing more than 115% IBW (12). This formula provides an adjusted weight that is larger than the adjusted weight given by Formula 2, with the rationale that patient compliance may be enhanced with more modest, stepwise alterations in nutrient intake (11). It is suggested to use this formula to calculate a starting point for prescribing energy needs, but then to periodically reassess weight and recalculate needs as the individual's status changes (11).

Formula 3 (5,12): Adjusted Weight (kg) = [(IBW – BW) × 0.25] + BW

Where:

BW = actual body weight
IBW = ideal body weight or standard body weight

Neither of these formulas has been validated, and the aims of the two formulas are slightly different. Formula 2 attempts to determine the weight that is added by the FFM from the fat tissue of an obese individual and adds this amount to the IBW. The energy needs based on the adjusted weight from Formula 2 approximate the amount of energy necessary to maintain the FFM of the individual, including the FFM contributed by the fat tissue. Formula 3 provides a weight that can be used to determine the level of energy that may be easier for the individual to maintain and is not based on FFM.

The two formulas can be used in a complementary fashion to best describe the needs and the most advantageous dietary prescription for an obese individual. Using Formula 2, the approximate level of energy needed to maintain weight can be determined from the adjusted weight. The adjusted weight from Formula 3 can then be used to determine an energy prescription that would be slightly higher and perhaps easier for the individual to maintain. The two results can be compared with the individual's actual intake, and an energy prescription that best meets the needs of the individual can be provided.

Example: For an individual with body weight of 187 lb (85 kg) and IBW of 132 lb (60 kg):

- Using Formula 2 and a mean of 0.22 and 0.33 for FFM factor:
  Adjusted weight = [(85 – 60) × (.275)] + 60 = (6.875) + 60 = 66.9 kg

  Energy needs based on 66.9 kg (× 35 kcal/kg) = 2,342 kcal

- Using Formula 3:
  Adjusted weight = [(60 – 85) × (.25)] + 85 = (–6.25) + 85 = 78.8 kg

  Energy needs based on 78.8 kg (× 35 kcal/kg) = 2,758 kcal

If the actual energy intake of the individual is close to 3,000 kcal, then it may be easier for the individual to achieve a prescription of 2,750 kcal (based on Formula 3). If, however, the actual energy intake is near 2,500 kcal, then an energy prescription of 2,300 (based on Formula 2) may be more prudent.

Determining protein requirements in obesity has not been addressed in the literature except in the issue of weight loss using very-low-calorie diets. Thus, there is no data regarding the optimal method for calculating maintenance protein needs in the obese individual. The rationale for adjusting body weight for protein is similar to that for adjusting for energy needs. As body weight increases, protein-containing tissues will also increase and an individual's protein requirements could be expected to increase as well. The degree to which protein needs would increase is not known, however. The increase may be proportional to the increase in FFM, but there is no data to support or refute this. For now, the NKF-K/DOQI Nutrition Guidelines recommend using the adjusted weight to determine protein needs in obese individuals.

There is currently no validated method for calculating energy and protein needs in the obese individual. Each person's nutrient needs must be assessed individually. In some situations, it may seem most appropriate to adjust body weight before determining energy or protein needs. In other situations, using actual body weight or IBW may seem more appropriate. The practitioner must use clinical judgment and expertise in determining the most appropriate method to use in assessing a particular individual's needs.

Adjustment for Underweight

The NKF-K/DOQI Nutrition Guidelines suggest adjusting IBW or SBW for individuals who are less than 95% IBW or SBW to better determine protein and energy requirements (12). Formula 3 can be used to provide an adjusted weight for underweight individuals (12). The practice of adjusting weight for determining protein and energy needs in individuals who are underweight is controversial and has not typically been used in the past. Currently, there is no research available which validates or disproves this approach. It is left to the practitioner to determine the appropriateness and usefulness of adjusting for underweight.

References

1. Olmstead Schulz L. Obese, overweight, desirable, ideal: where to draw the line in 1986? *J Am Diet Assoc.* 1986;86:1702–1704.

2. Kushner RF. Body weight and mortality. *Nutr Rev.* 1993;51:127–136.

3. Matarese LE, Gottschlich MM. *Contemporary Nutrition Support Practice: A Clinical Guide.* Philadelphia, Pa: WB Saunders; 1998.

4. Sichieri R, Everhart JE, Hubbard VS. Relative weight classifications in the assessment of underweight and overweight in the United States. *Int J Obes Relat Metab Disord.* 1992;16:303–312.

5. Kopple JD, Jones MR, Keshaviah PR, Bergstrom J, Lindsay RM, Moran J, Nolph KD, Teehan BP. A proposed glossary for dialysis kinetics. *Am J Kidney Dis.* 1995;26:963–981.

6. Frisancho AR. New standards of weight and body composition by frame size and height for assessment of nutritional status of adults and the elderly. *Am J Clin Nutr.* 1984;40:808–819.

7. World Health Organization. *Obesity: Preventing and Managing the Global Epidemic. Report of a WHO Consultation on Obesity, Geneva, 3–5 June 1997.* Geneva, Switzerland: WHO; 1998.

8. National Institutes of Health, National Heart, Lung, and Blood Institute. *Clinical Guidelines on the Identification, Evaluation, and Treatment of Overweight and Obesity in Adults.* Bethesda, Md: National Institutes of Health; 1998. NIH Publication No. 98–4083.

9. Meisler JG, St Jeor S. Summary and recommendations from the American Health Foundation's Expert Panel on Healthy Weight. *Am J Clin Nutr* 1996;63(Suppl):474S–477S.

10. National Kidney Foundation (NKF) Kidney Disease Outcome Quality Initiative (K/DOQI) Advisory Board. K/DOQI clinical practice guidelines for chronic kidney disease: evaluation, classification, and stratification. Guideline 6. Association of level of GFR with nutritional status. *Am J Kidney Dis.* 2002;39(2 Suppl 1): S128–S142.

11. McCann L, ed. *Pocket Guide to Nutrition Assessment of the Renal Patient.* 3rd ed. New York, NY: National Kidney Foundation; 2002.

12. National Kidney Foundation Kidney Disease Outcome Quality Initiative Advisory Board. K/DOQI clinical practice guidelines for nutrition in chronic renal failure. Appendix VII. Methods for performing anthropometry and calculating body measurements and reference tables. *Am J Kidney Dis.* 2000;35(6 Suppl 2):S76–S85.

13. National Center for Health Statistics. National Health and Nutrition Examination Survey: History. Available at: http://www.cdc.gov/nchs/about/major/nhanes/history.htm. Accessed April 28, 2002.

14. Flegal KM, Carroll MD, Ogden CL, Johnson CL. Prevalence and trends in obesity among US adults, 1999-2000. *JAMA.* 2002;288:1723–1727.

15. Flegal KM, Carroll MD, Kuezmarski RJ, Johnson CL. Overweight and obesity in the United States: prevalence and trends, 1960-1994. *Int J Obes Relat Metab Disord.* 1998;22:39–47.

16. Meisler JG, St Jeor S. Foreword for the American Health Foundation's Expert Panel on Healthy Weight. *Am J Clin Nutr.* 1996;63(Suppl):409S–411S.

17. National Center for Health Statistics Data Tables: Weight in pounds for males 20 years and over, number of examined persons, standard error of the mean, and selected percentiles, by race-ethnicity, age: United States, 1988–1994. Available at: http://www.cdc.gov/nchs/about/major/nhanes/wgtmal.pdf. Accessed November 8, 2002.

18. National Center for Health Statistics Data Tables: Weight in pounds for females 20 years and over, number of examined persons, standard error of the mean, and selected percentiles, by race-ethnicity, age: United States, 1988–1994. Available at: http://www.cdc.gov/nchs/about/major/nhanes/wgtfem.pdf. Accessed November 8, 2002.

19. Kopple JD, Zhu X, Lew NL, Lowrie EG. Body weight-for-height relationships predict mortality in maintenance hemodialysis patients. *Kidney Int.* 1999;56:1136–1148.

Section 4
Frame Size Determinations

To determine body frame size for use with ideal body weight (IBW) tables that specify small, medium, and large frame, one of two methods is normally used: wrist circumference or elbow breadth.

Method 1: Wrist Circumference

The subject's right wrist is measured with a narrow, nonstretchable centimeter tape measure. If the right wrist is affected by a fistula or arthritis, or has been broken, the left wrist is used. The measuring tape is placed above the smallest part of the wrist distal (toward the fingers) to the styloid process ("wristbone") (1). The tape should fit into the depression in front of the wristbone and touch the skin all around but not compress the soft tissue (1). Measurement is taken to the nearest 0.1 cm (1). The wrist circumference is used in the following formula, and the result is compared against the values in Table 4.1.

Formula 1 (2): $\text{Frame size} = \dfrac{\text{Height (cm)}}{\text{Wrist circumference (cm)}}$

Table 4.1   Frame Size Determined by Ratio of Height and Wrist Circumference

Frame Size	Males	Females
Small	> 10.4	> 11.0
Medium	9.6–10.4	10.1–11.0
Large	< 9.6	< 10.1
Reproduced from *Handbook of Total Parenteral Nutrition*, 2nd ed, with permission from Elsevier (2).		

Method 2: Elbow Breadth

The subject's arm is extended forward, perpendicular to the body, with the forearm bent upward at a 90° angle (1,3–5). The fingers are straight, and the back of the hand faces the measurer (4,5). While facing the subject, locate the two prominent bones on either side of the elbow (the lateral and medial epicondyles of the humerus) (1,3,4). Place the blades of the sliding caliper (blades pointing up) or the tips of the spreading caliper on the epicondyles (1). The caliper is held parallel or at a slight angle to the epicondyles and firm pressure is exerted to minimize the influence of soft tissue on the measurement (3,4). Measurements are made twice to the nearest 0.1 cm, and the mean of the two measurements is used (3). If calipers are not available, elbow breadth can be estimated by placing the thumb and index finger of one hand on the epicondyles and measuring the space between the fingers with a ruler or tape measure (1,3).

For the National Health and Nutrition Examination Survey (NHANES), three categories of frame size were established based on elbow breadth (5). "Small" frame size corresponds to less than the 15th sex- and age-specific percentile, "medium" frame size corresponds to between the 15th and 85th sex- and age-specific percentile, and "large" frame size corresponds to more than the 85th sex- and age-specific percentile of elbow breadth (5). These estimates of frame size are presented in Table 4.2.

Table 4.2   Frame Size by Elbow Breadth (cm) of US Male and Female Adults Derived from the Combined NHANES I and II Data Sets

Age (y)	Frame Size (cm)		
	Small	Medium	Large
Men			
18–24	≤ 6.6	> 6.6 and < 7.7	≥ 7.7
25–34	≤ 6.7	> 6.7 and < 7.9	≥ 7.9
35–44	≤ 6.7	> 6.7 and < 8.0	≥ 8.0
45–54	≤ 6.7	> 6.7 and < 8.1	≥ 8.1
55–64	≤ 6.7	> 6.7 and < 8.1	≥ 8.1
65–74	≤ 6.7	> 6.7 and < 8.1	≥ 8.1
Women			
18–24	≤ 5.6	> 5.6 and < 6.5	≥ 6.5
25–34	≤ 5.7	> 5.7 and < 6.8	≥ 6.8
35–44	≤ 5.7	> 5.7 and < 7.1	≥ 7.1
45–54	≤ 5.7	> 5.7 and < 7.2	≥ 7.2
55–64	≤ 5.8	> 5.8 and < 7.2	≥ 7.2
65–74	≤ 5.8	> 5.8 and < 7.2	≥ 7.2

The 10th and 90th percentiles, respectively, represent the predicted mean ±1.282 times the standard error (SE). Similarly, the 15th and 85th percentiles are the predicted mean minus and plus, respectively, 1.036 times the SE of the regression equation. There were significant differences in weight and body composition between black and white populations when age and height were considered. However, when the comparisons were made with reference to age, height, and frame size, there were only minor interpopulation differences. For this reason, all races (white, black, and others) included in the NHANES I and II surveys were merged for the purpose of calculating percentiles of anthropometric measurements.

Reproduced with permission by *The American Journal of Clinical Nutrition.* © 1984 Am J Clin Nutr. American Society for Clinical Nutrition (5).

References

1. Grant A, DeHoog S. *Nutritional Assessment and Support.* 5th ed. Seattle, Wash: Grant and DeHoog Publishers; 1999.

2. Grant JP. Nutritional assessment by body compartment analysis. In: *Handbook of Total Parenteral Nutrition.* 2nd ed. Philadelphia, Pa: WB Saunders; 1992:18–19.

3. Matarese LE, Gottschlich MM. *Contemporary Nutrition Support Practice: A Clinical Guide.* Philadelphia, Pa: WB Saunders; 1998.

4. Gibson RS. *Principles of Nutritional Assessment.* New York, NY: Oxford University Press; 1990.

5. Frisancho AR. New standards of weight and body composition by frame size and height for assessment of nutritional status of adults and the elderly. *Am J Clin Nutr.* 1984;40:808–819.

Section 5
Body Mass Index

The *body mass index* (BMI), also known as Quetelet's Index, is a method used to measure weight corrected for height. This index correlates highly with body fat and is useful for assessing weight status, obesity, and health risk (1). Studies have shown a relationship between BMI and morbidity and mortality in the general population, with relative risk of mortality increased for higher BMI levels (2,3).

Formula 1 (1): $\mathrm{BMI} = \dfrac{\mathrm{Wt\ (kg)}}{\mathrm{Ht\ (m^2)}}$

Where:

      Wt = body weight in kg
      Ht = height in meters

The following ranges for classification of weight using BMI (Table 5.1) are suggested by the World Health Organization's expert committee on obesity; the National Heart, Lung, and Blood Institute's (NHLBI) obesity clinical practice guidelines; the Dietary Guidelines for Americans; and Healthy People 2010 (4-8).

Table 5.1 Ranges for Classification of Weight Using BMI

BMI	Interpretation
< 18.5	Underweight—may be associated with health problems for some individuals (see below)
18.5–24.9	"Ideal" or healthy weight range—associated with lowest risk of illness and mortality for most people
25–29.9	Overweight—may be associated with health problems for some individuals
30–34.9	Class I Obesity—associated with increased risk of health problems such as heart disease, high blood pressure, and diabetes
35–39.9	Class II Obesity—associated with increased risk of health problems such as heart disease, high blood pressure, and diabetes
≥ 40	Class III Obesity—extreme obesity

There has been some disagreement about the type of association between a low BMI (< 18.5) and mortality risk (2,9,10). Some earlier studies on BMI showed an increased mortality risk with a lower BMI (2,9,11). These studies have been criticized for not controlling for smoking or coexisting disease, factors associated with both decreased weight and increased risk of mortality (2,9,11). Other studies that controlled for these factors have shown mixed results, with some studies indicating an increase in risk of mortality with a low BMI and others showing no change in the mortality risk with a low BMI (2,3, 9–12).

Dialysis

In the dialysis population, a different pattern of association between BMI and risk of mortality has been shown. In general, for patients on hemodialysis, higher weights and BMIs are not associated with an increase in morbidity and mortality as they are in the general population (13–16). In some cases, a decrease in risk of mortality or morbidity has been shown with increased BMI (13–15). In a group of 3,607 hemodialysis patients, Leavey et al found, after adjustment for smoking and coexistent disease, that risk of mortality increased with a BMI less than the population median of 23.9 and decreased with an increase in BMI more than 23.9 (13). The increased risk of mortality became significant as BMI decreased to less than approximately 19 (13). They also found that baseline BMI was predictive of mortality risk, independent of albumin and clinical assessment of nutritional status, even after 5 years (13). Kopple et al examined 1-year mortality rates in 12,965 hemodialysis patients and also discovered an increase in mortality risk with a low BMI and a decrease in mortality risk with higher BMI levels (15). The relative risk of death increased significantly for subjects below the 10th percentile for BMI of the population Kopple studied (18.8 for males and 18.4 for females) (15). It was also observed that the relative risk of death was significantly increased for subjects in the lower 50th percentile (less than 23.6 for males and 24.3 for females) vs those in the upper 50th percentile (15). In a sample of 7,719 US hemodialysis patients from the Dialysis Outcomes and Practice Patterns Study (DOPPS), patients with baseline BMIs less than 24.1 had a significantly higher risk of mortality than those with BMIs more than 28.1 (16). Furthermore, mortality risk significantly increased among patients with a decrease in BMI of more than 3.5% over a 6-month period (16).

Unlike the general population, there does not seem to be an "ideal" BMI range above and below which risk of morbidity and mortality increase for dialysis patients. The studies cited in the preceding paragraph indicate that there is a significant increase in mortality risk for dialysis patients with a low BMI, but the optimal BMI range is not known. Given the information available, the Kidney Disease Outcome Quality Initiative (K/DOQI) Clinical Practice Guidelines for Nutrition and for Chronic Kidney Disease have recommended that the BMI of hemodialysis patients be maintained in the upper 50th percentile, which would correspond to a BMI of at least 23.6 for males and 24.3 for females (17,18).

Transplantation

Among transplant recipients, it has been shown that higher pre-transplant BMI levels are associated with increased complications, graft failure, and mortality (19–23). In several smaller studies on transplant recipients, obese individuals with BMIs more than 30 had lower patient and graft survival rates up to 10 years post-transplant and more wound complications and cases of new-onset diabetes than the non-obese individuals (19,21–23). Additionally, a review of data on 16,110 male and 10,447 female transplant recipients showed a significant increase in the relative risk of graft failure as BMI increased to more than 27 in men and 33 in women (20). Because of the evidence for poorer outcome among obese patients, some investigators have recommended intervention for weight reduction to a BMI of less than 30 prior to transplantation (19,23).

BMI is not only helpful for assessing weight status but can also be used for determining "ideal" or "healthy" body weight (IBW) for an individual. Section 3 provides a method for finding IBW using BMI.

Amputation

BMI can be calculated in individuals with amputations by first calculating an *estimate of the full body weight* including the missing limb segments using Formula 2 (24). Section 17 provides a table of the percentage of total body weight contributed by certain segments of the body.

Formula 2: Estimated BW (kg) = $\dfrac{\text{measured weight (kg)}}{[100 - (\% \text{ weight of amputation}]} \times 100$

The *adjusted BMI* can then be calculated by substituting the estimated body weight in the equation for BMI (24).

Formula 3: $\text{BMI}_{\text{adj}} = \dfrac{\text{Estimated BW (kg)}}{\text{Ht (m}^2)}$

By substituting Formula 2 into Formula 3 for Estimated BW, the following formula is derived for calculating *adjusted BMI* (BMI_{adj}) directly:

Formula 4: $\text{BMI}_{\text{adj}} = \dfrac{\text{measured weight (kg)}}{\text{Ht (m}^2) \times [100 - (\% \text{ weight of amputation})]} \times 100$

Example: For a 5 ft 10 in (178 cm) male weighing 163 lb (74 kg) with a leg amputated to the knee:

The percentage of total body weight contributed by the missing limb = 1.5 (foot) + 4.4 (calf) = 5.9 percent

$$\text{Estimated BW(kg)} = \frac{74 \text{ kg}}{[100 - (5.9)]} \times 100 = \frac{74\text{kg}}{(94.1)} \times 100 = 78.6 \text{ kg}$$

$$\text{Adjusted BMI} = \text{BMI}_{\text{adj}} = \frac{78.6}{(1.78)^2} = 24.8$$

Or, adjusted BMI can be calculated using Formula 4:

$$\text{BMI}_{\text{adj}} = \frac{74}{(1.78)^2 \times [100 - (5.9)]} \times 100 = \frac{74}{(3.17) \times (94.1)} \times 100 = 24.8$$

References

1. Pi-Sunyer FX. Health implications of obesity. *Am J Clin Nutr.* 1991;53:1595S–1603S.

2. Kushner RF. Body weight and mortality. *Nutr Rev.* 1993;51:127–136.

3. Troiano RP, Frongillo EA, Sobal J, Levitsky DA. The relationship between body weight and mortality: a quantitative analysis of combined information from existing studies. *Int J Obes Relat Metab Disord.* 1996;20:63–75.

4. Seidell JC, Flegal KM. Assessing obesity: classification and epidemiology. *Br Med Bull.* 1997;53:238–252.

5. World Health Organization. Obesity: *Preventing and Managing the Global Epidemic. Report of a WHO Consultation on Obesity,* Geneva, 3–5 June 1997. Geneva, Switzerland: WHO; 1998.

6. *Nutrition and Your Health: Dietary Guidelines for Americans.* 5th ed. Washington, DC: US Depts of Agriculture and Health and Human Services; 2000. Home and Garden Bulletin No. 232.

7. *Clinical Guidelines on the Identification, Evaluation, and Treatment of Overweight and Obesity in Adults.* Bethesda, Md: National Institutes of Health, National Heart, Lung, and Blood Institute; 1998. NIH Publication No. 98–4083.

8. Food and Drug Administration and National Institutes of Health. *Healthy People 2010.* Vol II: *Nutrition and Overweight.* Pittsburgh, Pa: US Government Printing Office; 2001. Stock No. 017-001-00547-9.

9. Calle EE, Thun MJ, Petrelli JM, Rodriguez C, Heath CW. Body-mass index and mortality in a prospective cohort of US adults. *N Engl J Med.* 1999;341:1097–1105.

10. Sichieri R, Everhart JE, Hubbard VS. Relative weight classification in the assessment of underweight and overweight in the United States. *Int J Obes Relat Metab Disord.* 1991;16:303–312.

11. Stevens J. Impact of age on association between weight and mortality. *Nutr Rev.* 2000;58:129–137.

12. Stevens J, Cai J, Pamuk ER, Williamson DF, Thun MJ, Wood JL. The effect of age on the association between body-mass index and mortality. *N Engl J Med.* 1998;338:1–7.

13. Leavey SF, Strawderman RL, Jones CA, Port FK, Held PJ. Simple nutritional indicators as independent predictors of mortality in hemodialysis patients. *Am J Kidney Dis.* 1998;31:997–1066.

14. Fleischmann E, Teal N, Dudley J, May W, Bower JD, Salahudeen AK. Influence of excess weight on mortality and hospital stay in 1346 hemodialysis patients. *Kidney Int.* 1999;55:1560–1567.

15. Kopple JD, Zhu X, Lew NL, Lowrie EG. Body weight-for-height relationships predict mortality in maintenance hemodialysis patients. *Kidney Int.* 1999;56:1136–1148.

16. Pifer TB, McCullough KP, Port FK, Goodkin DA, Maroni BJ, Held PJ, Young EW. Mortality risk in hemodialysis patients and changes in nutritional indicators: DOPPS. *Kidney Int.* 2002;62:2238–2245.

17. National Kidney Foundation Kidney Disease Outcome Quality Initiative Advisory Board. K/DOQI clinical practice guidelines for nutrition in chronic renal failure. *Am J Kidney Dis.* 2000;35(6 Suppl 2):S1–S140.

18. National Kidney Foundation Kidney Disease Outcome Quality Initiative Advisory Board. K/DOQI clinical practice guidelines for chronic kidney disease: evaluation, classification, and stratification. *Am J Kidney Dis.* 2002;39(2 Suppl 2):S1–S246.

19. Pagenkemper JJ. Obesity: a serious risk factor in transplantation. *Nephrol News Issues.* 1999(Aug):58–62.

20. Chertow GM, Lazarus JM, Milford EL. Quetelet's index predicts outcome in cadaveric kidney transplantation. *J Ren Nutr.* 1996;6:134–140.

21. Holley JL, Shapiro R, Lopatin WB, Tzakis AG, Hakala TR, Starzl TE. Obesity as a risk factor following cadaveric renal transplantation. *Transplantation.* 1990;49:387–389.

22. Gill IS, Hodge EE, Novick AC, Steinmuller DR, Garred D. Impact of obesity of renal transplantation. *Transplant Proc.* 1993;25:1047–1048.

23. Modlin CS, Flechner SM, Goormastic M, Goldfarb DA, Papajcik D, Mastroianni B, Novick AC. Should obese patients lose weight before receiving a kidney transplant? *Transplantation.* 1997;64:599–604.

24. Himes JH. New equation to estimate body mass index in amputees. *J Am Diet Assoc.* 1995;95:646.

Section 6
Skinfold Measurements

Triceps and arm circumferences are easily accessible areas to measure body protein and fat. Reference data are not currently available specifically for the elderly or the dialysis population, but skinfold measurements can be useful for assessing long-term changes in subcutaneous fat and muscle stores in patients with chronic conditions (1,2). Standardization is extremely important for measurements to be valid. If different individuals perform measurements on the same patients, they should periodically standardize their techniques so they obtain similar values. Validity and reproducibility of the measurements is reduced in the very obese and in heavily muscled subjects.

Technique

- All measurements should be made in the patient's nonaccess-involved arm (or the right arm if there is an access in both arms) (2).
- Because hydration status can affect skinfold and circumference measures, measurements should be taken before the end of or after dialysis treatment (2).
- Measurement may be taken with the patient lying or sitting (2).
- Calipers should exert a constant pressure of 10 g/mm (2) and be accurate to 0.1 mm (3). They should be calibrated monthly with a calibration block.
- Calipers should be sanitized prior to each use.
- Measuring tape should be nonstretchable and preferably a disposable pediatric tape to avoid transmission of infection between patients.
- Values less than the 5th percentile for both arm muscle area and arm fat area indicate severe depletion (1,4). Values between the 5th and 10th percentiles for both arm muscle area and arm fat area represent moderate depletion (1,4). (See Tables 6.1 and 6.2.)

Procedure

Assessment of Upper Arm Midpoint

1. The subject's arm should be relaxed and bent at a 90° angle, palm up (1,3).
2. The observer should be behind the subject.
3. The disposable paper pediatric tape is positioned to measure the distance between the acromion process of the scapula (bony protrusion at lateral end of scapula ridge) and the olecron process (bony point of elbow) (1,3).
4. The halfway point is located and marked with a felt-tip pen.
5. The distance between the acromion process of the scapula and midpoint is read and recorded to the nearest 0.1 cm.

Measurement of Mid-Upper Arm Circumference (MAC)

1. The subject's arm should be relaxed, hanging by the subject's side.
2. The tape measure is looped loosely around the arm and positioned horizontally at the previously marked midpoint.
3. The tape measure is tightened around the contour of the arm, avoiding indentation or pinching (1).
4. The measurement is read and recorded to the nearest 0.1 cm (1,3).

Measurement of Triceps Skinfold (TSF)

1. The subject's arm should be relaxed, hanging by the subject's side.
2. The observer should remain behind the subject.
3. Using the left hand, the observer grasps a layer of skin and fat, approximately 1 cm above the previously marked midpoint, parallel to the long axis of the arm, then pulls it away from the underlying muscle (1,3,5). (If in doubt, the subject can contract and relax the arm muscles to ensure that no muscle is included in the pinch.)
4. The observer aligns the jaws of the calipers at the midpoint of the arm while maintaining a grip on the skinfold (1,3,5). The reading should be taken with the subject's arm relaxed.
5. The observer releases the arm of the caliper, waits approximately 3 seconds, and then takes another reading (3).
6. Three readings should be taken and the mean measurement recorded to the nearest 0.1 mm (1). Convert the mean measurement from millimeters to centimeters by dividing by 10.

Formulas

Calculations of *mid-upper arm fat area* (AFA) and *arm muscle area* (AMA) are based on measurements of MAC and TSF (5). Equations for estimating *AMA corrected for bone area* (AMA$_c$) are presented because they provide more accurate assessments of bone-free muscle area (1,6). These revised equations, however, have not been validated for use with elderly individuals and are not appropriate for obese patients (7). *It is essential to convert TSF to centimeters (cm) for the following equations.* Results are compared with the values in Tables 6.1 and 6.2.

Mid-Upper Arm Fat Area

Formula 1: $\text{AFA (cm}^2) = \dfrac{\text{MAC} \times \text{TSF}}{2} - \dfrac{\pi \times (\text{TSF})^2}{4}$

Mid-Upper Arm Muscle Area (5)

Formula 2: $\text{AMA (cm}^2) = \dfrac{[\text{MAC} - (\pi \times \text{TSF})]^2}{4\pi}$

Corrected AMA (6)

Formula 3: Men: $\text{AMA}_c \text{ (cm}^2) = \text{AMA} - 10$

Women: $\text{AMA}_c \text{ (cm}^2) = \text{AMA} - 6.5$

Table 6.1   Percentiles for Estimates of Mid-Upper Arm Fat Area (AFA) (cm2)*

Men	Percentiles								
Age (y)	5	10	15	25	50	75	85	90	95
18.0–24.9	5.5	6.9	7.7	9.2	13.9	21.5	26.8	30.7	37.2
25.0–29.9	6.0	7.3	8.4	10.2	16.3	23.9	29.7	33.3	40.4
30.0–34.9	6.2	8.4	9.7	11.9	18.4	25.6	31.6	34.8	41.9
35.0–39.9	6.5	8.1	9.6	12.8	18.8	25.2	29.6	33.4	39.4
40.0–44.9	7.1	8.7	9.9	12.4	18.0	25.3	30.1	35.3	42.1
45.0–49.9	7.4	9.0	10.2	12.3	18.1	24.9	29.7	33.7	40.4
50.0–54.9	7.0	8.6	10.1	12.3	17.3	23.9	29.0	32.4	40.0
55.9–59.9	6.4	8.2	9.7	12.3	17.4	23.8	28.4	33.3	39.1
60.0–64.9	6.9	8.7	9.9	12.1	17.0	23.5	28.3	31.8	38.7
65.0–69.9	5.8	7.4	8.5	10.9	16.5	22.8	27.2	30.7	36.3
70.0–74.9	6.0	7.5	8.9	11.0	15.9	22.0	25.7	29.1	34.9

Women	Percentiles								
Age (y)	5	10	15	25	50	75	85	90	95
18.0–24.9	10.0	12.0	13.5	16.1	21.9	30.6	37.2	42.0	51.6
25.0–29.9	11.0	13.3	15.1	17.7	24.5	34.8	42.1	47.1	57.5
30.0–34.9	12.2	14.8	17.2	20.4	28.2	39.0	46.8	52.3	64.5
35.0–39.9	13.0	15.8	18.0	21.8	29.7	41.7	49.2	55.5	64.9
40.0–44.9	13.8	16.7	19.2	23.0	31.3	42.6	51.0	56.3	64.5
45.0–49.9	13.6	17.1	19.8	24.3	33.0	44.4	52.3	58.4	68.8
50.0–54.9	14.3	18.3	21.4	25.7	34.1	45.6	53.9	57.7	65.7
55.9–59.9	13.7	18.2	20.7	26.0	34.5	46.4	53.9	59.1	69.7
60.0–64.9	15.3	19.1	21.9	26.0	34.8	45.7	51.7	58.3	68.3
65.0–69.9	13.9	17.6	20.0	24.1	32.7	42.7	49.2	53.6	62.4
70.0–74.9	13.0	16.2	18.8	22.7	31.2	41.0	46.4	51.4	57.7

*Reference data compiled from National Health and Nutrition Examination Survey (NHANES) I and II. Data are not specific for renal patients.

Adapted with permission from Frisancho AR. *Anthropometric Standards for the Assessment of Growth and Nutritional Status.* Ann Arbor, Mich: University of Michigan Press; 1990 (4).

Table 6.2 Percentiles for Estimates of Corrected Mid-Upper Arm Muscle Area (AMAc) (cm2)*

Men	Percentiles								
Age (y)	5	10	15	25	50	75	85	90	95
18.0-24.9	34.2	37.3	39.6	42.7	49.4	57.1	61.8	65.0	72.0
25.0-29.9	36.6	39.9	42.4	46.0	53.0	61.4	66.1	68.9	74.5
30.0-34.9	37.9	40.9	43.4	47.3	54.4	63.2	67.6	70.8	76.1
35.0-39.9	38.5	42.6	44.6	47.9	55.3	64.0	69.1	72.7	77.6
40.0-44.9	38.4	42.1	45.1	48.7	56.0	64.0	68.5	71.6	77.0
45.0-49.9	37.7	41.3	43.7	47.9	55.2	63.3	68.4	72.2	76.2
50.0-54.9	36.0	40.0	42.7	46.6	54.0	62.7	67.0	70.4	77.4
55.9-59.9	36.5	40.8	42.7	46.7	54.3	61.9	66.4	69.6	75.1
60.0-64.9	34.5	38.7	41.2	44.9	52.1	60.0	64.8	67.5	71.6
65.0-69.9	31.4	35.8	38.4	42.3	49.1	57.3	61.2	64.3	69.4
70.0-74.9	29.7	33.8	36.1	40.2	47.0	54.6	59.1	62.1	67.3

Women	Percentiles								
Age (y)	5	10	15	25	50	75	85	90	95
18.0-24.9	19.5	21.5	22.8	24.5	28.3	33.1	36.4	39.0	44.2
25.0-29.9	20.5	21.9	23.1	25.2	29.4	34.9	38.5	41.9	47.8
30.0-34.9	21.1	23.0	24.2	26.3	30.9	36.8	41.2	44.7	51.3
35.0-39.9	21.1	23.4	24.7	27.3	31.8	38.7	43.1	46.1	54.2
40.0-44.9	21.3	23.4	25.5	27.5	32.3	39.8	45.8	49.5	55.8
45.0-49.9	21.6	23.1	24.8	27.4	32.5	39.5	44.7	48.4	56.1
50.0-54.9	22.2	24.6	25.7	28.3	33.4	40.4	46.1	49.6	55.6
55.9-59.9	22.8	24.8	26.5	28.7	34.7	42.3	47.3	52.1	58.8
60.0-64.9	22.4	24.5	26.3	29.2	34.5	41.1	45.6	49.1	55.1
65.0-69.9	21.9	24.5	26.2	28.9	34.6	41.6	46.3	49.6	56.5
70.0-74.9	22.2	24.4	26.0	28.8	34.3	41.8	46.4	49.2	54.6

*Values have been adjusted for bone area by subtracting 10.0 cm^2 for men and 6.5 cm^2 for women from the calculated mid upper arm muscle area.

Reference data compiled from National Health and Nutrition Examination Survey (NHANES) I and II. Data are not specific for renal patients.

Adapted with permission from Frisancho AR. *Anthropometric Standards for the Assessment of Growth and Nutritional Status*. Ann Arbor, Mich: University of Michigan Press; 1990 (4).

References

1. Matarese LE, Gottschlich MM. *Contemporary Nutrition Support Practice: A Clinical Guide*. Philadelphia, Pa: WB Saunders; 1998.

2. Chumlea WC. Anthropometric assessment of nutritional status in renal disease. *J Ren Nutr*. 1997;7:176–181.

3. Grant A, DeHoog S. *Nutritional Assessment and Support*. 5th ed. Seattle, Wash: Grant and DeHoog Publishers; 1999.

4. Frisancho AR. *Anthropometric Standards for the Assessment of Growth and Nutritional Status*. Ann Arbor, Mich: University of Michigan Press; 1990.

5. Frisancho AR. New norms of upper limb fat muscle areas for assessment of nutritional status. *Am J Clin Nutr*. 1981;34:2540–2545.

6. Heymsfield SB, McManus CB, Smith J, Stevens V, Nixon DW. Anthropometric measurement of muscle mass: revised equations for calculating bone-free arm muscle area. *Am J Clin Nutr*. 1982;36:680–690.

7. Gibson RS. *Principles of Nutritional Assessment*. New York, NY: Oxford University Press; 1990.

Section 7
Subjective Global Assessment

Assessment of nutritional status involves many factors, such as laboratory results, anthropometric measurements, and diet and weight history. *Subjective Global Assessment* (SGA) is a relatively new method that relies on the clinician's expertise and experience to subjectively rate a patient's nutritional status based on medical history and physical exam. It has been used and validated in several patient populations, including chronic kidney disease (CKD) patients (1–4), and is recommended by the National Kidney Foundation Kidney Disease Outcome Quality Initiative (NKF-K/DOQI) Clinical Practice Guidelines for Nutrition in Chronic Renal Failure as a valid and clinically useful measure of protein-energy nutritional status in maintenance dialysis patients (5).

The components of SGA, which have all been incorporated separately in *Guidelines for Nutrition Care of Renal Patients,* 3rd ed, are (6–9):

1. *Weight Change:* The amount and rate of weight loss and its pattern during the previous 6 months.
2. *Dietary Intake:* A historical review of the patient's dietary intake with comparison of the usual and recommended intake to the current dietary intake.
3. *Gastrointestinal Symptoms:* Determination of any significant gastrointestinal symptoms lasting at least 2 weeks in duration. Symptoms can include anorexia, nausea, vomiting, and/or diarrhea.
4. *Functional Capacity:* Changes in the patient's energy or activity levels that are related to nutritional status.
5. *Metabolic Demands:* The metabolic demands of the patient's underlying disease state and any acute stresses that may alter metabolic demands (eg infection, fever, surgery).
6. *Physical Signs:* Assessment for loss of subcutaneous fat, muscle wasting, and/or fluid retention. Physical symptoms suggestive of nutrient-specific deficiencies are sometimes also included (eg, glossitis, cheilosis). A guide for evaluating nutrient-specific deficiencies is provided in Section 12.

Based on subjective weighting of these features, the patient is classified as well nourished, moderately malnourished, or severely malnourished. Guides have been developed to assist the clinician in performing and rating the SGA, and a comprehensive review of the methodology, including example forms, has been published in the literature (6,10).

References

1. Baker JP, Detsky AS, Wesson DE, Wolman SL, Stewart S, Whitewell J, Langer B, Jeejeebhoy KN. Nutritional assessment: a comparison of clinical judgment and objective measurements. *New Engl J Med.* 1982;306:969–972.

2. Detsky AS, McLaughlin JR, Baker JP, Johnston N, Whittaker S, Mendelson RA, Jeejeebhoy KN. What is subjective global assessment of nutritional status? *JPEN J Parenter Enteral Nutr.* 1987;11:8–13.

3. Hasse J, Strong S, Gorman MA, Liepa G. Subjective global assessment: alternative nutrition-assessment technique for liver transplant candidates. *Nutrition.* 1993;9:339–343.

4. Enia G, Sicuso C, Alati G, Zoccali C. Subjective global assessment of nutrition in dialysis patients. *Nephrol Dial Transplant.* 1993;8:1094–1098.

5. National Kidney Foundation Kidney Disease Outcome Quality Initiative Advisory Board. K/DOQI clinical practice guidelines for nutrition in chronic renal failure. Guideline 9. Subjective global nutritional assessment (SGA). *Am J Kidney Dis.* 2000;35(6 Suppl 2):S30–S31.

6. McCann L. Subjective global assessment as it pertains to the nutritional status of dialysis patients. *Dial Transplant.* 1996;25:190–199,202,225.

7. Jeejeebhoy KN, Detsky AS, Baker JP. Assessment of nutritional status. *JPEN J Parenter Enteral Nutr.* 1990;14:193S–196S.

8. Manning EMC, Shenkin A. Nutritional assessment in the critically ill. *Crit Care Clin.* 1995;11:603–634.

9. McCann L, ed. *Pocket Guide to Nutrition Assessment of the Renal Patient.* 3rd ed. New York, NY: National Kidney Foundation; 2002.

10. McCann L, Yates L, Ezaki-Yamaguchi J, Akiyama P. Forms to monitor and assess nutritional status of renal patients. *J Ren Nutr.* 1995;5:151–155.

Section 8
Laboratory Values in Dialysis Patients

Many factors can affect the interpretation of laboratory values, including accuracy and precision of the test, laboratory methodology, diurnal variation, infection, hormonal status, disease state, hemolysis, and many others. In dialysis patients, certain factors occur more frequently, and some of these and their implications for interpretation are discussed in this section.

General Factors

Day of the Week

Monthly laboratory testing is typically done on a specified day of the week at each facility. Some facilities draw labs on the first dialysis day of the week (usually after a longer interdialytic period) and some draw midweek (usually after a shorter interdialytic period). Results and interpretation of the results will vary depending on the day of the draw, ie the length of the interdialytic period prior to the draw. Laboratory indexes that are high in renal patients because of renal disease (eg, BUN, creatinine, phosphorus) will typically be higher for the first of the week lab draw due to the extra time allowed for these substances to accumulate. Other laboratory indexes may be lower (eg, sodium) due to increased hydration levels.

Hydration Status

As mentioned above, hydration status can affect laboratory values because of the influence on serum concentration. Because hydration status can vary widely in dialysis patients, both between patients and within a particular patient, this should always be considered in the interpretation of laboratory values in this patient population.

Time of Day

Some laboratory indexes vary with the time of day due to individual diurnal variation. They may also vary because of differences in food consumption throughout the day, and in relation to the time of dialysis (1). The dialysis patient who has had blood drawn in the evening likely has been consuming food during the day, and possibly a large meal prior to dialysis (in contrast to patients in the early-morning shift), and thus might be absorbing significant amounts of water and solute, thereby influencing laboratory results (1). Typically, a patient receives dialysis on a regular schedule at the same time of day, so if a patient changes to a different time of day, it should be noted that there may be some alteration in the patient's laboratory levels.

Blood Draw Methodology

The methodology used for drawing blood can sometimes affect results. The techniques and timing used in drawing blood samples and in processing the samples need to be consistent to assure accurate results. Hemolysis, contamination of a specimen, or dilution of a specimen can be caused by errors in blood sampling (2). In particular, blood specimens for BUN measurement can be sensitive to sampling errors, such as incorrect timing of sample collection, and need to be drawn in a certain manner so that dialysis adequacy can be calculated accurately and results interpreted correctly (2–4). Pre-dialysis BUN should be measured before dialysis begins and without dilution of the blood sample (3,4). Post-dialysis BUN should be measured after dialysis ends and after access recirculation has resolved (3,4). The National Kidney Foundation Kidney Disease Outcomes Quality Initiative (NKF-K/DOQI) Clinical Practice Guidelines for Hemodialysis Adequacy clearly define an acceptable methodology for BUN sampling (4).

Specific Tests

Albumin

It has been shown that the two most common laboratory methods used for determining serum albumin levels have different results in dialysis patients (5,6). Bromcresol green (BCG) and bromcresol purple (BCP) dyes are typically used to measure albumin levels. In individuals with normal renal function, BCP is usually the accepted method because it more nearly agrees with nephelometry, the gold-standard method for albumin measurement (5). However, in several studies with dialysis patients, the BCP method consistently resulted in lower values than BCG or nephelometry (5,6). There is no consensus on which method is preferential, but in most guidelines, including those used by the Centers for Medicare & Medicaid Services (CMS) (formerly known as the Health Care Financing Administration [HCFA]) and the ESRD networks, the albumin level represented is based on the BCG method. In a facility that uses the BCP method, the BCP albumin level corresponding to the BCG level will be approximately 0.5 mg/dL less.

Albumin levels are decreased by conditions that promote an acute-phase response, such as infection or trauma (7). Dialysis patients frequently experience infections and/or surgery, and thus may have reduced albumin levels in response to these stresses. In addition to investigating possible nutritional causes of a decreased albumin, recent infections, surgeries, and illnesses should also be investigated as possible contributors.

Calcium

Normally, 46% to 50% of total calcium is ionized with most of the remainder (40%) bound to proteins (8). The ionized calcium is the physiologically active form that the body uses, but because of cost and availability issues, total calcium typically is measured. Unfortunately, total calcium values are affected by hypoalbuminemia, a state that is common in renal patients, whereas ionized calcium values are not affected by albumin status. In patients with decreased serum albumin, the total calcium value will decrease but the ionized calcium level will not (8,9). Total calcium may be adjusted for a decreased serum albumin to better reflect the amount of biologically active calcium, but the appropriate use of this correction and the interpretation of the results is controversial (9). Adjustment of total calcium levels provides only an *estimate* of the amount of active calcium that is present in the blood. Laboratory-calculated ionized calcium levels are also not accurate in hypoalbuminemia (8). If a true value is required, then ionized calcium should be measured directly.

Adjustment of total calcium can be useful clinically for detecting possible calcium disorders. For example, in cases of severe hypoalbuminemia, "normal" total calcium levels would actually indicate highly elevated ionized calcium levels. The high ionized calcium may not be detected unless total calcium levels were adjusted for hypoalbuminemia. To adjust for low albumin levels, the total calcium level needs to be adjusted upward by 0.8 mg/dL for every 1 g/dL decrease in albumin (8,9). Thus, for a patient whose albumin level drops from 4.0 g/dL to 3.0 g/dL, a total calcium level of 9.0 mg/dL at the lower albumin level would correspond to a total calcium level of 9.8 mg/dL at the higher albumin level. As stated before, because this is only an approximation, measuring ionized calcium levels directly is more accurate.

Acidosis and alkalosis can also affect calcium levels (8,9). Adjustment formulas for acidosis and alkalosis are available for situations when serum albumin levels are normal. These formulas are presented here, but they have not been tested in renal patients and are not typically used in this population. They are provided for interest only. In the case of acidosis, more calcium is ionized (8,9). Thus, total calcium is adjusted upward by 2 mg/dL for each 0.1 decrease in pH (9). Conversely, in alkalosis the ionized fraction of calcium is decreased, and thus the total calcium is adjusted downward by 2 mg/dL for each 0.1 increase in pH (8,9). Again, if the true physiologically active form of calcium needs to be known, ionized calcium should be measured directly.

Parathyroid Hormone

Different assays have been used to assess the parathyroid hormone (PTH) level: intact, C-terminal, and N-terminal. The C-terminal assay measures the biologically inactive C-terminal fragment of the PTH molecule as well as the intact PTH (via the C-terminal end). The N-terminal assay measures the biologically active N-terminal fragment of the PTH molecule as well as the intact PTH (via the N-terminal end). In dialysis patients, the preferred methodology is the intact PTH assay (i-PTH), which measures the biologically active molecule with both C- and N-terminals intact (10–13). Recently it has been discovered, however, that the i-PTH assay also measures some N-terminally-truncated PTH fragments that do not include the entire 84 amino acids of the intact PTH molecule (10–13). These fragments, referred to as non-(1–84) PTH, are usually excreted by the kidneys but accumulate in patients with decreased renal function (10,13). Experiments have shown that one or more of these fragments can modify bone cell activity and skeletal remodeling, leading to speculation that these fragments may contribute to the skeletal resistance to PTH seen in renal failure (12,13). A new assay, known as the Whole PTH or (1–84) PTH assay, is available and seems to detect only the intact PTH molecule and none of the non-(1–84) PTH fragments (10–12). Comparisons of PTH levels measured by the Whole PTH assay and the traditional i-PTH assay show approximately 40% to 50% lower PTH levels with the Whole PTH assay (11,12). Only a few studies have been completed using the Whole PTH assay, so data to guide interpretation of results are sparse (12). It is still to be determined if the Whole PTH assay will provide more reliable information for the diagnosis of hyperparathyroidism and bone disease (11,12). Further studies are needed before the Whole PTH assay can be applied in the clinical setting (12).

References

1. Mattana J, Patel A, Wagner JD, Maesaka JK, Singhal PC. Effect of time of day of dialysis shift on serum biochemical parameters in patients on chronic hemodialysis. *Am J Nephrol.* 1995;15:208–216.

2. Beto JA, Bansal VK, Kahn S. The effect of blood draw methodology on selected nutritional parameters in chronic renal failure. *Adv Renal Repl Ther.* 1999;6:85–92.

3. Beto JA, Bansal VK, Ing TS, Daugirdas JT. Variation in blood sample collection for determination of hemodialysis adequacy. *Am J Kidney Dis.* 1998;31:135–141.

4. NKF-K/DOQI clinical practice guidelines for hemodialysis adequacy: update 2000. *Am J Kidney Dis.* 2001;37(1 Suppl 1):S7–S64.

5. Zazra JJ. Biochemical markers of nutrition: technical aspects. *J Ren Nutr.* 1997;7:65–68.

6. Wick MJ, Wilkens K, Moritz J. Albumin testing methods differ: implications for the dialysis patient. *Dial Transplant.* 1994;23:282–283,286.

7. Yeun JY, Kaysen GA. Factors influencing serum albumin in dialysis patients. *Am J Kidney Dis.* 1998;32(6, Suppl 4):S118–S125.

8. Chernecky CC, Berger BJ, eds. *Laboratory Tests and Diagnostic Procedures*. 2nd ed. Philadelphia, Pa: WB Saunders; 1997.

9. Matarese LE, Gottschlich MM. *Contemporary Nutrition Support Practice: A Clinical Guide*. Philadelphia, Pa: WB Saunders; 1998.

10. Avram MM. Risks and monitoring of elevated parathyroid hormone in chronic renal failure (a review). *Dial Transplant*. 2001;30:147–155.

11. Slatopolsky E, Finch J, Clay P, Martin D, Sicard G, Singer G, Gao P, Cantor T, Dusso A. A novel mechanism for skeletal resistance in uremia. *Kidney Int*. 2000;58:753–761.

12. Goodman WG, Jüppner H, Salusky IB, Sherrard DJ. Parathyroid hormone (PTH), PTH-derived peptides, and new PTH assays in renal osteodystrophy. *Kidney Int*. 2003;63:1–11.

13. Brossard JH, Yamamoto LN, D'Amur P. PTH metabolites in renal failure: bioactivity and clinical implications. *Semin Dial*. 2002;15:196–201.

Bibliography

Craven D, Moreschi J. A dietitian-driven protocol for the management of renal bone disease in hemodialysis patients. *J Ren Nutr*. 1996;6:105–109.

Ikizler TA. Biochemical markers: clinical aspects. *J Ren Nutr*. 1997;7:61–64.

Kaysen GA, Stevenson FT, Depner TA. Determinants of albumin concentration in hemodialysis patients. *Am J Kidney Dis*. 1997;29:658–668.

Kopple JD, Massry SG, eds. *Nutritional Management of Renal Disease*. Baltimore, Md: Williams & Wilkins; 1997.

Section 9
Energy Estimation

Basal energy expenditure (BEE) is defined as the energy expenditure of a healthy person at full repose, before or immediately upon awakening, prior to eating or engaging in any activity (1). It is slightly lower than resting energy expenditure (REE), although the terms BEE and REE are often used interchangeably. REE is considered equal to BEE plus the thermogenic effect of feeding and possibly a small activity factor (1).

The most common equation for determining BEE is the Harris-Benedict equation, published in 1919 (2). Studies in recent years have reported that the Harris-Benedict equation overestimates energy requirements, and other equations have been proposed (3–7). The Harris-Benedict equation, however, seems to predict energy needs as closely as some of these equations (8) and continues to be the most widely used in clinical and research settings.

Formula 1: Harris-Benedict Equations

Males: BEE (kcal/day) = 66.47 + 13.75 (Wt) +5.00 (Ht) − 6.76 (Age)

Females: BEE (kcal/day) = 655.1 + 9.56 (Wt) +1.85 (Ht) − 4.68 (Age)

Where:
Wt = weight in kg
Ht = height in cm
Age = age in years

To determine actual energy needs, BEE is multiplied by activity and stress factors:

Formula 2: Energy needs = BEE × Activity factor × Stress factor(s)

Table 9.1   Activity Factors

Activity	Factor
Confined to bed	1.2
Out of bed/ambulatory	1.3

Table 9.2   Stress Factors

Stress	Factor
Non-dialyzed chronic kidney disease	1.0
Maintenance dialysis	1.0
Maintenance transplant	0.9–1.0
Fever	1.0 + 0.13 per °C > 37°C
Surgery:	
Minor/uncomplicated	1.0–1.2
Major/complicated	1.1–1.4
Skeletal/blunt trauma	1.15–1.35
Infections:	
Mild	1.0–1.2
Moderate	1.2–1.4
Severe/sepsis	1.4–1.6
Burns:	
< 20% burn surface area (BSA)	1.0–1.5
20–40% BSA	1.5–1.85
> 40% BSA	1.85–2.0
Malnutrition (severe)	0.6–0.8

Energy needs can also be determined based on weight. Nitrogen balance studies in chronic kidney disease (CKD) patients have assessed the energy intake needed to maintain a positive nitrogen balance when the recommended protein level is consumed. These studies form the basis for the weight-based energy recommendations. The National Kidney Foundation Kidney Disease Outcome Quality Initiative (K/DOQI) Nutrition and Chronic Kidney Disease committees have made recommendations for CKD (predialysis and dialysis) patients based on these studies, and these recommendations are included in Table 9.3 (9,10).

Table 9.3   Energy Needs for Patients with CKD

Condition	Energy needs (kcal/kg)
CKD (predialysis and dialysis):	
< 60 years old	35
≥ 60 years old	30–35
Acute renal failure	30–40 (best determined through use of indirect calorimetry)
Transplant:	
Acute phase	30–35
Chronic phase	25–35 (to maintain an appropriate weight)

Age, activity level, fitness level, and body composition are all factors that influence metabolic rate and energy needs. These factors need further investigation to determine the extent and direction of the effects. For obese individuals, weight is often adjusted before determining energy needs. Section 3 discusses the rationale and methods for adjusting body weight in obesity.

References

1. Matarese LE, Gottschlich MM. *Contemporary Nutrition Support Practice: A Clinical Guide.* Philadelphia, Pa: WB Saunders; 1998.

2. Harris JA, Benedict FG. A Biometric Study of Basal Metabolism in Man. Washington, DC: Carnegie Institute; 1919. Publication No. 279.

3. Mifflin MD, St Jeor ST, Hill LA, Scott BJ, Daugherty SA, Koh YO. A new predictive equation for resting energy expenditure in healthy individuals. *Am J Clin Nutr.* 1990;51:241–247.

4. Owen OE, Holup JL, D'Alessio DA, Craig ES, Polansky M, Smalley KJ, Kavle EC, Bushman MC, Owen LR, Mozzoli MA, Kendrick ZV, Boden GH. A reappraisal of the caloric requirements of men. *Am J Clin Nutr.* 1987;46:875–85.

5. Owen OE, Kavle E, Owen RS, Polansky M, Caprio S, Mozzoli MA, Kendrick ZV, Bushman MC, Boden G. A reappraisal of caloric requirements in healthy women. *Am J Clin Nutr.* 1986;44:1–19.

6. Cunningham JJ. Body composition as a determinant of energy expenditure: a synthetic review and a proposed general prediction equation. *Am J Clin Nutr.* 1991;54:963–969.

7. Fredrix EWHM, Soeters PB, Deerenberg IM, Kester ADM, von Meyenfeldt MF, Saris WHM. Resting and sleeping energy expenditure in the elderly. *Eur J Clin Nutr.* 1990;44:741–747.

8. Taaffe DR, Thompson J, Butterfield G, Marcus R. Accuracy of equations to predict basal metabolic rate in older women. *J Am Diet Assoc.* 1995;95:1387–1392.

9. National Kidney Foundation Kidney Disease Outcome Quality Initiative Advisory Board. K/DOQI clinical practice guidelines for nutrition in chronic renal failure. Guideline 17: daily energy intake for maintenance dialysis patients. *Am J Kidney Dis.* 2000;35(6 Suppl 2):S44–S45.

10. National Kidney Foundation Kidney Disease Outcome Quality Initiative Advisory Board. K/DOQI clinical practice guidelines for chronic kidney disease: evaluation, classification, and stratification. Guideline 9. Association of level of GFR with nutritional status. *Am J Kidney Dis.* 2002;39(2 Suppl 1):S128–S142.

Bibliography

Cataldo CB, Rolfes SR, Whitney EN. *Understanding Clinical Nutrition.* St Paul, Minn: West Publishing; 1991.

Grant A, DeHoog S. *Nutritional Assessment and Support.* 5th ed. Seattle, Wash: Grant and DeHoog Publishers; 1999.

Harris JA, Benedict FG. *A Biometric Study of Basal Metabolism in Man.* Washington, DC: Carnegie Institute of Washington; 1919.

Kopple JD, Massry SG, eds. *Nutritional Management of Renal Disease.* Baltimore, Md: Williams & Wilkins; 1997.

Long CL, Schaffel N, Geiger JW, Schiller WR, Blakemore WS. Metabolic response to injury and illness: estimation of energy and protein needs from indirect calorimetry and nitrogen balance. *JPEN J Parenter Enteral Nutr.* 1979;3:452–456.

Mahan LK, Escott–Stump S, eds. *Krause's Food, Nutrition, and Diet Therapy.* 10th ed. Philadelphia, Pa: WB Saunders; 2000.

McCann L, ed. *Pocket Guide to Nutrition Assessment of the Renal Patient.* 3rd ed. New York, NY: National Kidney Foundation; 2002.

Monson P, Mehta RL. Nutrition in acute renal failure: a reappraisal for the 1990s. *J Ren Nutr.* 1994;4:58–77.

Stover J, ed. *A Clinical Guide to Nutrition Care in End–Stage Renal Disease.* 2nd ed. Chicago, Ill: American Dietetic Association; 1994.

Section 10
Intradialytic Parenteral Nutrition

Intradialytic Parenteral Nutrition (IDPN) is a noninvasive method of administering intravenous nutritional support to hemodialysis patients. The IDPN solution is infused directly into the venous drip chamber of the hemodialysis machine during dialysis treatment. Because IDPN is delivered only during the dialysis treatment, it does not provide complete nutrition support for a patient and cannot meet total nutritional needs. If a patient is unable to receive sufficient energy and protein via the gastrointestinal route to adequately supplement the IDPN, total parenteral nutrition (TPN) should be considered (1).

Indications for Use

It is difficult to define specific indications or circumstances in which IDPN is the treatment of choice for malnourished hemodialysis patients (1). Criteria for initiating and discontinuing IDPN have been suggested by one author (2). Medicare has developed certain guidelines for reimbursement of outpatient parenteral nutrition (IDPN and TPN). If a patient's method of reimbursement is Medicare, specific criteria must be met for the patient to qualify for IDPN. In general, a clinical picture that depicts malnutrition in the presence of malabsorption may need to be supported. If malnutrition exists despite nutrition counseling, supplement use, and attempts to correct medical issues that may be affecting nutritional status, then IDPN is considered the next step.

The goals for using IDPN are improved albumin levels, prevention of continued weight loss or weight gain, increased intake, and improved quality of life (ie, decreased hospitalizations, decreased infections, wound healing, increased energy) (3–5).

IDPN Components and Administration

The IDPN solution consists of IV dextrose, amino acids, and sometimes lipids. The total volume of solution infused should be based on the patient's weight, interdialytic weight gains, time on dialysis, and other factors that affect fluid removal tolerance. Infusion rates should not exceed 350 mL/hour due to the absence of studies confirming the safety of higher rates of administration (6).

Dextrose Component

- The dextrose component of IDPN should provide enough carbohydrate substrate to prevent the oxidation of amino acids for energy (7).
- The amount of dextrose provided should be based on patient weight and length of the dialysis treatment. The maximal oxidative rate for glucose is estimated at 3 to 6 mg/kg/minute, however there are some estimates as high as 9 mg/kg/minute. Total parenteral nutrition is typically restricted to these rates to avoid lipogenesis and a respiratory quotient more than 1.0 (7–8). However, in

contrast to TPN, IDPN is only provided for a short time period (3 to 4 hours, 3 times a week), and thus a higher rate of delivery (eg, up to 8 mg/kg/minute) may be tolerated (5).

- Because dialysis patients rarely require additional free water, the most concentrated form of dextrose (70% dextrose or D70) is recommended.
- If it is determined that the total grams of carbohydrate should be decreased, the strategy should be to decrease the amount of dextrose in the IDPN solution by reducing the volume of D70, not the concentration (7).

Amino Acid Component

- Mixed amino acid solutions containing essential and nonessential amino acids are used, generally providing 1.0 to 1.5 g protein per kg body weight (5,7).
- Although some of the amino acids are removed by the dialysis process, approximately 90% of the amino acids provided by IDPN are retained (7,9).
- As with dextrose, the most concentrated form of amino acids is generally used to avoid additional free water (ie, 15% amino acids).

Lipid Component

- The energy contribution of lipids should be maximized, but should not exceed 2.5 g/kg/day (9).
- It is recommended that no more than 50 g of lipids (250 cc of 20% or 500 cc of 10%) be administered in a 4-hour period (5). This correlates to a maximum rate of 62.5 cc/hour for 20% and 125 cc/hour for 10% (7).
- To avoid fat overload, lipids should not provide more than 60% of the total energy, and triglyceride levels should be monitored (9).
- The initial solution of IDPN usually does not contain lipids, allowing overall tolerance to the infusion to be established (9). This also makes it easier to determine the cause of an allergic reaction if it occurs when lipid infusion begins.
- For the patient who has never before received lipids, a test dose should be given and the patient should be monitored during the first 30 minutes of lipid infusion to detect any allergic or adverse reactions (7).
- Patients with known allergies to eggs should not receive lipid solutions (8). Lipids are also contraindicated in patients with severe hypertriglyceridemia (8).
- Lipid infusion may be given as long as pretreatment triglyceride levels remain less than 500 mg/dL and infusion of lipids does not increase lipids more than 50% (see Monitoring Guidelines to follow).

Formulas for Calculating Grams of Nutrients and Energy Provided

Grams of Carbohydrate and Energy from Dextrose

Formula 1: Carbohydrates (g) = Volume × Concentration

Where:

        Volume (cc) = volume of dextrose solution
        Concentration = decimal representation of dextrose concentration (ie 0.50 for D50%)

Formula 2: Energy (kcal) = Carbohydrate (g) × 3.4

Grams of Protein and Energy from Amino Acids

Formula 3: Protein (g) = Volume × Concentration

Where:

Volume (cc) = volume of amino acid solution

Concentration = decimal representation of amino acid concentration (ie 0.15 for 15% amino acids)

Formula 4: Energy (kcal) = Protein (g) × 4.0

Grams of Fat and Energy from Lipids

Formula 5: Fat (g) = Volume × Concentration

Where:

Volume (cc) = volume of lipid solution

Concentration = decimal representation of lipid concentration (ie 0.10 for 10% lipids, 0.20 for 20% lipids)

Formula 6: For 10% lipids: Energy (kcal) = Fat (g) × 1.1

For 20% lipids: Energy (kcal) = Fat (g) × 2.0

Monitoring Guidelines

- Blood glucose levels are checked before treatment, 1 hour into the treatment, and post-treatment (1,7). If levels are elevated during the hemodialysis procedure (ie, glucose ≥ 300 mg/dL), IV insulin should be given (1,6,9). The postdialysis blood glucose goal is 200 to 300 mg/dL (1,6). If the post-dialysis blood glucose level is less than 200 mg/dL, an additional 30 to 60 g oral simple carbohydrate is provided to the patient and blood glucose levels are rechecked before the patient leaves the dialysis unit (6).
- Serum triglyceride levels should be evaluated before the first and second consecutive IDPN treatment days with lipid-containing solutions to check liver clearance (6–9). If the second level is more than 50% more than the first level, the patient may not be effectively clearing lipids from the circulation (7). Long-term tolerance is checked by monitoring serum liver function tests, cholesterol, and triglycerides on a monthly basis (1,6,7).
- Hypophosphatemia may occur if the patient is subject to "refeeding syndrome," and can be treated by adding either potassium phosphate or sodium phosphate to the IDPN solution (1,6).
- If hypokalemia is noted, either potassium may be added to the IDPN solution or the potassium concentration of the dialysate may be increased (1).
- Abnormal intradialytic cramping may be indicative of hyponatremia or excessive fluid removal (1,6). If the patient is hyponatremic, it is suggested that normal saline may be administered or that 70 to 150 mEq sodium chloride may be added to the IDPN formula (1,5,6).

Table 10.1 presents the initial and routine monitoring recommendations for IDPN. Monitoring more frequently than monthly may be indicated if a problem occurs.

Table 10.1 Frequency of Monitoring of Laboratory and Nutritional Data—Intradialytic Parenteral Nutrition (IDPN) Therapy

| Obtain Baseline | Predialysis | First Treatments (frequency as stated below) | | | Monthly |
		1 hour	Postdialysis	2 Weeks	
BUN, creatinine					X
Albumin					X
Sodium					X
Potassium	X*			X	X
Phosphorus	X*			X	X
Calcium	X*				X
Serum glucose	X†	X†	X†		X
Cholesterol					X
Triglycerides	X‡				X
Liver enzymes					X
Kt/V (or URR)				X	X

*These tests should be done for the first 3 infusions of IDPN, then monitored as indicated.
†These tests should be done for the first 6 infusions of IDPN. The need for and frequency of blood glucose tests should be reassessed at that time.
‡This test should be done prior to the first and second infusions that contain lipids.

References

1. Foulks CJ. Intradialytic parenteral nutrition. In: Kopple JD, Massry SG, eds. *Nutritional Management of Renal Disease*. Baltimore, Md: Williams & Wilkins; 1997.

2. Lazarus JM. Recommended criteria for initiating and discontinuing intradialytic parenteral nutrition therapy. *Am J Kidney Dis*. 1999;33:211–216.

3. McQuiston B, Potempa L, Deguzman LG, Sackmann S. Intradialytic parenteral nutrition efficacy: a retrospective study. *J Ren Nutr*. 1997;7:102–105.

4. Cano N, Labastie-Coeyrehourq J, Lacombe P, Stroumza P, de Costanzo-Dufetel J, Durbec JP, Coudray-Lucas C, Cynober L. Perdialytic parenteral nutrition with lipids and amino acids in malnourished hemodialysis patients. *Am J Clin Nutr*. 1990;52:726–30.

5. Cato Y. Intradialytic parenteral nutrition therapy for the malnourished hemodialysis patient. *J Intraven Nurs*. 1997;20:130–135.

6. Goldstein DJ, Strom JA. Intradialytic parenteral nutrition: evolution and current concepts. *J Ren Nutr*. 1991;1:9–22.

7. Fresenius Medical Care/NMC Homecare. *Comprehensive Renal Nutrition Support Program: IDPN/IPN Clinical Manual*. Lexington, Mass: Fresenius Medical Care/NMC Homecare; 1998.

8. Matarese LE, Gottschlich MM. *Contemporary Nutrition Support Practice: A Clinical Guide*. Philadelphia, Pa: WB Saunders; 1998.

9. Stover J, ed. *A Clinical Guide to Nutrition Care in End-Stage Renal Disease*. 2nd ed. Chicago, Ill: American Dietetic Association; 1994.

Section 11

Vitamins and Minerals in Chronic Kidney Disease

Research has shown that vitamin and mineral needs of patients with chronic kidney disease (CKD) are as individualized as other nutrient needs. Ideally, the dietitian should evaluate the vitamin and mineral needs of each client individually rather than recommend standard supplements or restrictions. Vitamin and mineral status should be part of a renal patient's regular, complete, nutrition assessment.

To assess the vitamin and mineral status of a CKD patient adequately, the dietitian needs to collect and evaluate appropriate medical, dietary, and biochemical data unique to the patient's clinical presentation. Based on these data, the dietitian should determine the individual patient's need for supplementation and/or diet modification.

The following steps outline a suggested procedure for assessing vitamin and mineral status:

1. Collect a complete diet history and evaluate for nutrient adequacy based on the current Dietary Reference Intakes (DRIs) and recommendations specific for renal failure.
2. Obtain laboratory data on tissues and serum vitamin and mineral stores and compare against the appropriate standards. The laboratory and clinical methodologies used for measuring and assessing biochemical data should be considered in this evaluation.
3. Determine whether dialysis losses, malabsorption, or retention of vitamins and minerals is occurring.
4. Evaluate concurrent medical conditions for possible influences on vitamin or mineral status.
5. Assess medications and their effect on vitamin and mineral status.

Individualizing and monitoring a CKD patient's vitamin and mineral status should be a goal of treatment, but it also requires time and resources. In some situations, recommending DRI levels of water-soluble vitamins may be a prudent step. Assessment of other nutrients, including fat-soluble vitamins, minerals, trace minerals, and other substances, requires an in-depth nutrition assessment and evaluation of biochemical data.

Fat-Soluble Vitamins

Studies do not support routine supplementation of fat-soluble vitamins other than vitamin D for patients consuming well-balanced, adequate diets. Evaluation for deficiency and supplementation with the appropriate vitamins may be indicated for patients with malabsorption conditions or other risk factors as noted.

Vitamin A

The risk of vitamin A toxicity continues to be a controversial topic. Data from the Third National Health and Nutrition Examination Survey (NHANES III) have shown that serum vitamin A levels increase significantly with increasing serum creatinine levels in the US population, and numerous studies have shown elevated levels of vitamin A in the liver and plasma of CKD (predialysis, hemodialysis, and peritoneal dialysis) patients (1–3). However, plasma carotenoid levels have been reported to be markedly reduced and symptoms related to vitamin A toxicity are not usually seen in CKD (predialysis and dialysis) patients because most of the vitamin is bound to protein and thus not active (2,4). Comprehensive reviews of vitamin A metabolism and implications in renal disease have been published (1,5).

The general recommendation is that vitamin A should not be routinely supplemented in patients with CKD (predialysis and dialysis). Vitamin A levels are elevated in transplant recipients as well, and supplementation of vitamin A is not recommended (2,5). Clinical experience indicates that low serum levels of vitamin A may be more an indicator of malnutrition than depleted vitamin A status. Thus, encouraging an overall increase in nutrient content of the diet may be the recommended mode of treatment. If vitamin A supplements are used, however, the supplemental dose of vitamin A should not be larger than the DRI for normal healthy adults (700–900 µg/day) (5). Because patients with nephrotic syndrome may lose protein-bound vitamins, a daily intake of the DRI for vitamin A may be indicated (5). In patients with acute renal failure, specific recommendations are not well defined. Vitamin A supplements are probably not necessary unless patients are on TPN, and then no more than the DRI for vitamin A should be given (5,6). For patients with CKD (predialysis) who chronically ingest less than two-thirds of the DRI for vitamin A, a vitamin A supplement (not to exceed the DRI) may be prescribed (5).

Vitamin D

The form of vitamin D that is obtained from the diet or produced in the skin must be hydroxylated in the liver and in the kidney to be converted to its most biologically active form (5,7–9). This activated form of vitamin D, 1,25 dihydroxycholecalciferol [$1,25(OH)_2D_3$] or calcitriol, plays a substantial role in the interactions among calcium, phosphorus, parathyroid hormone (PTH), and bone metabolism. Calcitriol aids in the absorption of calcium and phosphorus in the gastrointestinal (GI) tract, inhibits PTH formation and secretion, and stimulates activity of osteoclasts in the bone (2,5,7,8,10). These actions all contribute to an increase in serum calcium and phosphorus (2,5,7,8,10). When renal function deteriorates, production of calcitriol decreases, resulting in an increase in PTH secretion and a decrease in calcium absorption (2,5,8,10,11). Hyperphosphatemia associated with renal failure will also inhibit calcitriol production, and acidosis and the accumulation of uremic toxins may reduce calcitriol levels as well (2,7,10,12–16). The low serum calcitriol levels contribute to the hyperparathyroidism and hypocalcemia seen with renal failure and the associated bone disease that frequently develops. To help increase calcium levels, reduce PTH levels, and prevent the development of bone disease, supplementation of calcitriol is frequently provided to dialysis patients and is sometimes utilized in CKD (predialysis) patients (5,10).

Supplementation with calcitriol in CKD (predialysis and dialysis) patients will depend on serum calcium, phosphorus, and PTH levels. These levels should be monitored closely to avoid any complications from calcitriol use (8). Calcitriol will increase calcium and phosphorus absorption from the GI tract and can aggravate hypercalcemia and hyperphosphatemia (8,13,17–20). Hypercalcemia and a high calcium-phosphorus product (Ca x P) can lead to soft tissue and cardiovascular calcification (19,21–24). The risks of hypercalcemia and metastatic and cardiovascular calcifications increase with the use of calcitriol in conjunction with calcium-based binders and supplements (8,15,21,25–27).

Overuse of calcitriol can lead to oversuppression of PTH and promote the development of adynamic bone disease (8,11,16,27). The low bone turnover in adynamic bone disease decreases the bone's ability to buffer calcium and phosphorus levels in the blood, and the result can be hypercalcemia and hyperphosphatemia (8,16,21).

New vitamin D analogs have been developed that suppress PTH levels while having less effect on serum calcium levels (8,16,19,28). In the United States, two analogs, paricalcitol (19-nor-1,25 dihydroxyvitamin D_2) and doxercalciferol (1α,25 dihydroxyvitamin D_2), are currently approved by the Food and Drug Administration (FDA) and are in use (8,16,19). These vitamin D analogs may allow for better control of calcium, phosphorus, and PTH levels and help prevent bone disease and the occurrence of metastatic calcifications.

After renal transplantation, the synthesis of calcitriol is usually restored (2,5,10). However, hyperparathyroidism present before transplantation may remain, often leading to bone loss (2,5,29). Immunosuppressants can exacerbate existing bone disease and lead to increased bone turnover and further bone loss (2,5,29). Supplementation with vitamin D, along with adequate calcium intake, can help minimize the long-term metabolic bone complications after transplantation (2,5,29). Transplant recipients should receive at least the DRI of vitamin D (5–15 mg/day or 200–600 IU/day) via diet or supplements to help maintain adequate calcium levels (5). Serum and urinary calcium levels, PTH levels, and bone density studies may be obtained to monitor the effectiveness of treatment for bone disease (5).

Vitamin E

Studies of vitamin E status in CKD (predialysis and dialysis) patients have shown varying results, with serum levels of vitamin E reported to be decreased, normal, and increased (2,5). Vitamin E supplementation in renal failure is generally not considered necessary except in the case of patients receiving TPN, during which supplementation in the amount of 10 IU/day (7 mg/day) is recommended (5). Because of the antioxidant properties of vitamin E, supplementation of 10 IU/day (7 mg/day) is also commonly suggested for the general renal population. High doses of vitamin E may help improve lipid peroxidation, but these higher levels may also interfere with vitamin K–dependent coagulation factors and inhibit platelet aggregation (2,5,30). Supplementation of vitamin E at 400 to 600 IU/day (265 to 400 mg/day) has been shown to decrease the incidence and severity of leg cramps in dialysis patients (31,32). Again, caution should be taken and patient clotting monitored closely when using these high doses.

Vitamin E–coated dialyzers have been developed to help protect against oxidative stress in hemodialysis patients (33,34). The hemodialysis procedure is associated with the development of oxidative stress and may disturb the body's ability to protect against oxygen free radicals (34). Repeated contact between the hemodialysis patient's blood and the dialyzer membrane stimulates the production of oxygen free radicals, even when dialysis membranes with improved biocompatibility are used (33,34). Vitamin E–coated dialyzers have been shown to improve the oxidative stress associated with hemodialysis (33,34). Serum levels of vitamin E seem to remain unchanged (33).

Vitamin K

Vitamin K supplements are not routinely recommended for patients with CKD. If a patient is receiving antibiotics and eating poorly, particularly for extended periods of time, supplementation of 10 mg/day vitamin K may be beneficial to help prevent a deficiency (5). It is recommended to routinely provide patients receiving TPN with 7.5 mg/week of vitamin K (5). Because of its role in the coagulation cascade, however, supplementation with vitamin K can lead to increased clotting and can counteract the effects of anticoagulation therapy (5). Patients on anticoagulation therapy who are receiving vitamin K supplementation should have clotting times monitored closely.

Adequate levels of vitamin K are essential for maintaining bone health (5,35). Decreased bone density and increased risk of bone fractures have been associated with depressed vitamin K levels in the general population (5,35). In hemodialysis patients, one study found an increased risk of fractures and hyperparathyroidism with suboptimal vitamin K status (35). Further research is needed, however, to determine whether vitamin K supplementation may aid in the prevention or treatment of renal bone disease (5).

Water-Soluble Vitamins

Because of increased losses of water-soluble vitamins in the dialysate, supplementation of water-soluble vitamins at or near the level of the DRI is typically recommended for dialysis patients. In patients with high urine output receiving dialysis, patients with diarrhea or vomiting, patients with poor dietary intake, or patients with medical complications, evaluation for deficiency and additional supplementation of water-soluble vitamins may be indicated.

Vitamin C

Decreased vitamin C levels have been shown to be significantly associated with increased serum creatinine levels in the US population (3), with CKD (predialysis) patients demonstrating low vitamin C levels (2,5). In acute renal failure, hemodialysis, and peritoneal dialysis patients, there is some risk for vitamin C deficiency because of a combination of insufficient intake and dialysate losses (5,36). However, excess intake of vitamin C in CKD patients may contribute to an increased risk of hyperoxalemia, which can lead to an increased deposition of oxalate in bone and soft tissue (5,36–41). The current recommendation for CKD (predialysis and dialysis) and acute renal failure patients is 60 to 100 mg/day of vitamin C, but no more unless dietary evaluation and evidence of an increased requirement is documented in an individual patient (2,5,36).

Thiamin (Vitamin B-1)

Dietary sources of thiamin include legumes, whole-grain foods, nuts, seeds, and various meats, and thus a diet low in protein and/or potassium may result in a reduced intake of thiamin. Approximately 10% of CKD (predialysis) patients following a low-protein diet (0.6 mg/kg/day) will become thiamin deficient (2). Peritoneal dialysis patients also often exhibit low serum thiamin levels (2). Serum thiamin levels tend to be normal in hemodialysis patients, however (2,5). In spite of these normal levels, the activity of the thiamin-dependent transketolase enzyme in erythrocytes has been reported to be insufficient in more than 50% of hemodialysis patients (2,5,42). Peritoneal patients also have been shown to have decreased erythrocyte transketolase activity (2). This insufficiency, though, may be due to an inhibition of the enzymatic system rather than an actual vitamin deficiency (42). Because serum levels of thiamin are frequently normal in hemodialysis patients, and because parameters of thiamin deficiency seem to be readily corrected with small doses of thiamin hydrochloride, it is recommended that CKD (predialysis and dialysis) patients receive a supplement of 1.5 mg/day in addition to the thiamin contained in the food consumed (5,36). For patients with acute renal failure, 1.5 to 2.0 mg/day of thiamin is recommended to compensate for poor intake and increased losses from dialysis (2,5).

Riboflavin (Vitamin B-2)

Plasma riboflavin levels are typically normal or high in dialysis patients, and a deficiency does not seem common in maintenance dialysis patients (5,42). Because riboflavin supplements are safe and because riboflavin deficiency may occur in dialysis patients who are eating poorly, a daily supplement equal to the DRI (1.1–1.3 mg/day) has been recommended (5). CKD (predialysis) patients on a low-protein diet (0.6 g/kg/day) may exhibit decreased riboflavin levels because low-protein diets are often inadequate in riboflavin (2,5). It is recommended to supplement CKD (predialysis) patients with 1.8 mg/day of riboflavin (5). Because of reduced intake and losses of water-soluble vitamins in the dialysate, it is recommended that acute renal failure patients be supplemented with up to 2.0 mg/day of riboflavin (2,5).

Niacin (Vitamin B-3)

Little data are available regarding niacin status in patients with renal failure. Because niacin is quickly removed metabolically from plasma, losses in dialysate are expected to be low (5). Because a low-protein diet may provide a low amount of niacin and because niacin deficiency has been shown to occur in some dialysis patients, recommendations are that CKD (predialysis and dialysis) patients take between

14 and 20 mg of supplemental niacin per day (comparable to the DRI) (2,5,36). Supplementation of 14 to 20 mg/day of niacin is also recommended for acute renal failure patients (2,5).

Folate

Although dietary intake among CKD (predialysis and dialysis) patients is often below the DRI for folate, the incidence of folate deficiency is rare and hemotologic manifestations of folate deficiency are uncommon (5). Plasma folate levels have been reported to be normal (43–45). Folate is significantly cleared or lost during high-efficiency dialysis, however, which may lead to reduced folate levels (46).

The need for folate supplementation in patients with CKD is controversial, but folate supplements seem safe for CKD (predialysis and dialysis) patients, with only mild side effects (nausea, headache, vivid dreams) reported in some cases using higher doses (2,5,47).

With folate supplementation, though, there is a potential for masking the hematologic disturbances associated with vitamin B-12 deficiency (5). Patients using folate supplements should have vitamin B-12 levels checked or be prescribed vitamin B-12 supplements to avoid the risk of neurologic manifestations of vitamin B-12 deficiency (48–50). The standard recommendation for folate supplementation in CKD (predialysis and dialysis) and acute renal failure patients is 1.0 mg/day (5).

Recently, the association between plasma homocysteine and vascular disease has received much attention, and this association has been shown to exist in the CKD population (5,44,45,47). Folate supplementation reduces homocysteine levels in the normal population and has also been shown to reduce homocysteine levels in CKD patients, including transplant patients (2,5,45,47–62). Reductions in homocysteine of approximately 30% have been realized in dialysis patients using folate supplements of 0.5 to 15.0 mg/day, but this reduction is not sufficient to normalize homocysteine levels (47–49,52,55,58,60). Transplant patients may respond better to folate supplementation, as evidenced by a larger percentage achieving normal homocysteine levels (56,57). The National Kidney Foundation Task Force on Cardiovascular Disease recently issued a report containing recommendations for treatment of hyperhomocysteinemia in the renal population (63). The report recommends 5 mg/day of folate, along with vitamins B-6 (50 mg/day) and B-12 (400 µg/day), to reduce homocysteine levels and possibly protect against vascular disease in CKD (predialysis, dialysis, and transplant) patients (63). Comprehensive reviews of the interactions of folate and homocysteine in the renal population are available for further review (45,64,65).

Pyridoxine (Vitamin B-6)

Biochemical deficiency of the coenzyme pyridoxal-5'-phosphate (PLP), the active form of vitamin B-6, has been identified in CKD (predialysis and dialysis) patients (5,36,42,66–69). This may be due in part to decreased dietary intake, losses through dialysis, altered phosphorylation of pyridoxal on PLP, and increased metabolic clearance of PLP in CKD (predialysis and dialysis) patients (5,6,64,70). Tobacco smoking decreases plasma vitamin B-6 levels, and many common medications interfere with the actions or metabolism of vitamin B-6 (5). Diabetes has also been associated with an increased risk of vitamin B-6 deficiency in dialysis patients, and use of erythropoietin (EPO) may increase the requirement of vitamin B-6 because of increased erythropoiesis (66,70). Additionally, use of high-efficiency dialysis can increase losses of vitamin B-6 (2,46,69). Vitamin B-6 deficiency may be linked with increased concentrations of plasma and tissue oxalate in CKD patients (5). Elevated oxalate levels can lead to calcium oxalate deposits in tissues and organs (5).

The need for supplementation of vitamin B-6 in dialysis patients is widely recognized (5,36, 42,64,67,70). In general, to correct for vitamin B-6 deficiency, it is recommended that adult hemodialysis and peritoneal dialysis patients receive supplementation of 10 mg/day of pyridoxine HCl (2,5,6,36, 64,69). A supplement of 10 mg/day pyridoxine HCl is also recommended for patients with acute renal failure to correct vitamin B-6 deficiency (5). Data is lacking about the need for supplemental vitamin

B-6 in CKD (predialysis and transplant) patients, but 5 mg/day is commonly seen as a recommendation for CKD (predialysis) patients (5).

In CKD (predialysis and dialysis) patients, the ability to excrete metabolites of vitamin B-6 may be impaired (5). Peripheral neuropathy has been reported with doses of more than 200 mg/day pyridoxine over long periods (5,47). Doses of pyridoxine of more than 100 mg/day should be used cautiously when prescribed for extended periods of time (5).

In the general population and in patients with CKD, decreased vitamin B-6 levels may be associated with elevated plasma homocysteine (5,44,48,64,66). The benefit of vitamin B-6 supplementation to decrease homocysteine levels in CKD patients is unclear. Several reports indicate no effect of vitamin B-6 supplements on reducing serum homocysteine levels (45,51,53,54). One study, however, found that there may be a modest effect when vitamin B-6 is used in conjunction with folate in hemodialysis patients but not CKD (predialysis) patients (68). Nevertheless, many of the recent studies that have looked at reducing homocysteine levels with vitamin therapy have included anywhere from 10 mg to 200 mg per day of vitamin B-6 (49,55–57,68,71). The National Kidney Foundation Task Force on Cardiovascular Disease has recommended a dose of 50 mg/day of vitamin B-6, in addition to folate (5 mg/day) and vitamin B-12 (400 µg/day), to reduce homocysteine levels in CKD (predialysis, dialysis, and transplant) patients (63).

Cobalamin (vitamin B-12)

Studies have reported normal to high plasma levels of vitamin B-12 in CKD (predialysis, dialysis, and transplant) patients (5,42,44,45,50). Vitamin B-12 is protein-bound and expected to exhibit little loss during dialysis (2,5,6,36,50,64). Because vitamin B-12 is found primarily in animal-food sources, patients who avoid all animal foods may have an inadequate intake of vitamin B-12 and should be evaluated for possible deficiency (72,73). Absorption of vitamin B-12 relies on intrinsic factor (IF), a glycoprotein produced by the gastric mucosa (72,73). Inadequate production or secretion of IF can result in vitamin B-12 malabsorption and deficiency and can lead to pernicious anemia (72,73). A patient with atropic gastritis or partial or total gastrectomy may lose production of IF and is thus at risk for vitamin B-12 deficiency (72,73). Absorption of vitamin B-12 occurs in the ileum, and ileal disease or surgical resection can also lead to vitamin B-12 malabsorption (72,73). Patients with vitamin B-12 deficiency due to malabsorption may require periodic vitamin B-12 injections.

Because vitamin B-12 intake has been found to be less than the DRI in some dialysis patients, and because of vitamin B-12's importance in red blood cell synthesis along with folate and iron, a daily supplement comparable to the DRI (2–3 µg/day) has been recommended for CKD (predialysis and dialysis) patients (2,5,36). A daily supplement of 2 to 3 µg/day of vitamin B-12 is also recommended for patients with acute renal failure (2,5). Patients prescribed folate supplementation should be provided vitamin B-12 supplements whenever vitamin B-12 levels cannot be established to avoid the risk of neuropathy (48-50). Folate supplementation may mask any hemotologic signs of vitamin B-12 deficiency, but neurologic degeneration that can occur with vitamin B-12 deficiency will not be corrected (5,50,72).

The role of vitamin B-12 in reducing homocysteine levels in CKD patients has not been clarified. Reports have shown mixed results, with some indicating a small benefit from use of vitamin B-12 in addition to folate, and others finding no benefit (2,45,50,54,55,59,74). Several studies evaluating the potential of vitamin therapy in reducing homocysteine have used oral vitamin B-12 supplements in the treatment regimens, with amounts ranging from 400 to 1000 µg/day (49,50,55–57,69,71). It has been suggested that the limited oral bioavailability of vitamin B-12 may prevent achievement of high enough levels to affect homocysteine levels (50,75). One study showed a significant reduction in homocysteine levels in hemodialysis patients with the addition of parenteral vitamin B-12 (75). The recommendation by the National Kidney Foundation Task Force on Cardiovascular Disease is that 400 µg /day of vitamin B-12 be prescribed, along with folate and vitamin B-6, to reduce homocysteine levels in CKD (predialysis, dialysis, and transplant) patients (63).

Biotin

Biotin levels have been reported to be in the normal range or higher in CKD patients (2,36,42). However, because some cases of biotin deficiency have been reported in hemodialysis patients, and because biotin intake in CKD (predialysis) patients consuming low-protein diets has been reported to be less than the DRI, the current recommendation is to supplement biotin at an amount of 30 to 100 µg/day (1–3 times the DRI of 30 µg/day) in CKD (predialysis and dialysis) patients (5). It is suggested that acute renal failure patients receive 200 µg/day of biotin (5).

Pantothenic Acid

Levels of pantothenic acid are frequently normal, and no evidence of pantothenic acid deficiency has been seen in CKD patients, although data on this vitamin in the renal population are sparse (5). The DRI for pantothenic acid has been set at 5 mg/day, and based on experimental data in humans, it seems to be both potentially beneficial and safe to recommend supplementation of pantothenic acid in CKD (predialysis and dialysis) patients at this level (2,5). Because of potential for decreased intake and dialysis losses of water-soluble vitamins, a dose of 10 mg/day of pantothenic acid is recommended for acute renal failure patients (5).

Table 11.1 presents DRIs for vitamins, as well as vitamin supplementation recommendations for patients with end-stage renal disease.

Table 11.1   Vitamin Supplementation Recommendations in Chronic Kidney Disease

Nutrient	US DRI[a] (adults >18 yrs)	Predialysis	Hemodialysis	Peritoneal Dialysis	Acute Renal Failure (TPN)
Vitamin A	**700–900 µg /day**	None	None	None	See text
Vitamin D	5–15 µg/day*	Individualized	Individualized	Individualized	Unknown
Vitamin E	**15 mg/day (22 IU/day)**	See text	See text	See text	10 IU/day (7 mg/day)
Vitamin K	90–120 µg/day*	None[b]	None[b]	None[b]	7.5 mg/week
Vitamin C	**75–90 mg/day**	60–100 mg/day	60–100 mg/day	60–100 mg/day	60–100 mg/day
Thiamine (B–1)	**1.1–1.2 mg/day**	1.5 mg/day	1.5 mg/day	1.5 mg/day	1.5–2.0 mg/day
Ribofalvin (B–2)	**1.1–1.3 mg/day**	1.8 mg/day	1.1–1.3 mg/day	1.1–1.3 mg/day	2.0 mg/day
Niacin	**14–16 mg/day**	14–20 mg/day	14–20 mg/day	14–20 mg/day	14–20 mg/day
Folate	**0.4 mg/day**	1.0 mg/day[c]	1.0 mg/day[c]	1.0 mg/day[c]	1.0 mg/day
Pyridoxine (B–6)	**1.3–1.7 mg/day**	5 mg/day[c]	10 mg/day[c]	10 mg/day[c]	10 mg/day
Cobalamin (B–12)	**2.4 µg/day**	2–3 µg/day[c]	2–3 µg/day[c]	2–3 µg/day[c]	3 µg/day
Biotin	30 µg/day*	30–100 µg/day	30–100 µg/day	30–100 µg/day	200 µg/day
Pantothenic Acid	5 mg/day*	5 mg/day	5 mg/day	5 mg/day	10 mg/day

[a]DRI levels represent Recommended Dietary Allowances (RDA) and Adequate Intakes (AI). RDAs are in listed **bold type** and AIs are listed in ordinary type followed by an asterisk (*).
[b]Supplementation of vitamin K may be needed for patients who are not eating and who receive antibiotics (5).
[c]Higher levels may be indicated to reduce plasma homocysteine levels. See text.

Minerals

Patients with CKD experience alterations in mineral metabolism. Mineral levels must be monitored and supplemented or restricted as indicated by appropriate evaluation techniques.

Phosphorus

Serum phosphorus levels are influenced by serum calcium, vitamin D, and parathyroid hormone (PTH) levels and the kidney's ability to excrete and reabsorb phosphorus (2,5,17). In mild renal insufficiency, serum phosphorus levels usually remain normal despite loss of renal function (2,5,17,76). This is due to an increase in the fractional excretion of phosphorus in response to increased PTH levels (2,5,17). As GFR decreases below 30 to 40 mL/min/1.73m^2, however, the kidney is no longer able to sufficiently eliminate phosphorus, and hyperphosphatemia usually develops (5,17). High serum phosphorus levels reduce serum calcium, suppress vitamin D production, and lead to an increase in PTH (both directly and secondary to the lower calcium and vitamin D levels) (2,5,15,19,76–78). Hyperphosphatemia is also associated with metastatic calcification, increased blood pressure, and cardiovascular complications, and has been shown to be directly related to increased relative mortality risk in patients with CKD (17,19,22,24,79–83). A recent study found that patients with phosphorus levels more than 6.5 mg/dL had a 27% higher relative mortality risk than patients with phosphorus levels less than 5.5 mg/dL (81). High phosphorus levels contribute to an increased calcium-phosphorus product (Ca x P) and Ca x P levels more than 72 are also associated with an increase in relative risk of mortality (81). Cardiac calcification and calcific uremic arteriolopathy (otherwise known as calciphylaxis) have been shown to occur with Ca x P levels between 55 and 65 (19,22,24). Because of the increased risks of metastatic calcification, cardiovascular disease, and death with high phosphorus and Ca x P product, Block and Port have recommended that serum phosphorus levels be maintained between 2.5 and 5.5 mg/dL and Ca x P be maintained at less than 55 (19). Other authors have suggested even lower limits, recommending that phosphorus levels be kept at less than 5.0 mg/dL and Ca x P less than 50 to 55 (16,83).

In CKD patients, phosphorus intake generally needs to be reduced, and sometimes "phosphate binders," medications that bind phosphorus in the digestive tract and limit phosphorus absorption, need to be used to maintain appropriate phosphorus levels (2). Hemodialysis is not efficient at removing phosphorus from the blood, and the quantity of phosphorus removed is less than that required to avoid severe hyperphosphatemia (5,18,77,84). Peritoneal dialysis may be more efficient at removing phosphorus, but it usually cannot remove a sufficient quantity either (5,18,77,84,85). Thus, in dialysis patients, a dietary restriction of phosphorus is usually necessary (2,5,18,76,83). Because protein foods are high in phosphorus, maintaining an adequate protein intake in dialysis patients also limits the ability to restrict phosphorus intake (19,86). Phosphate binders are often required to maintain serum phosphorus levels at an acceptable level (2,5,18,76,83).

Hyperphosphatemia can result despite dietary phosphate restriction and phosphate binder compliance. Inadequate dialysis, severe hyperparathyroidism, variability in dissolution rates among phosphate binders, treatment with EPO, in vitro hemolysis, and extreme hypertriglyceridemia have all been cited as additional causes or contributors to hyperphosphatemia (18,19,76,77,83,87–89). In addition, acidosis can cause a shift of phosphorus from inside the cell, leading to elevated serum phosphorus levels (88). Spurious (pseudo) hyperphosphatemia may also be seen in cases of multiple myeloma (myeloma proteins bind phosphate and interfere with the colorimetric measurement of serum phosphate) (88).

Hypophosphatemia is common after renal transplantation, and often phosphorus supplements are needed temporarily (2,5,90). Hypophosphatemia can also occur in CKD (predialysis and dialysis) patients. Patients taking excessive amounts of phosphate binders or other phosphate-binding medications, such as milk of magnesia, may experience low phosphorus levels. Hypophosphatemia may occur after a parathyroidectomy for correction of hyperparathyroidism (ie, hungry-bone syndrome) or in cases of active alcoholism (88,91).

Acute renal failure patients often are unable to excrete phosphorus adequately and may experience hyperphosphatemia (2,5,92). Hypophosphatemia may also be seen in CKD patients receiving parenteral nutrition support, and may also occur as a result of refeeding syndrome or diuretic therapy (2,88,92). Serum phosphorus levels should be monitored frequently in these patients, and phosphorus intake individualized based on serum levels (2,5,92).

Calcium

Hypocalcemia is often seen in CKD (predialysis and dialysis) and acute renal failure patients due to 1) hyperphosphatemia from decreased renal phosphorus excretion, 2) deficiency of vitamin D, which results in decreased intestinal absorption of calcium, and 3) skeletal resistance to the action of PTH, resulting in a decreased release of calcium from the bone (2,5,11,85,93,94). Foods high in calcium are also generally restricted because of their high phosphorus content, leading to a decreased dietary intake of calcium (5,95).

To achieve appropriate calcium levels and balance, supplementation with calcium and/or vitamin D is often required (2,5,95–97). Calcium-containing phosphate binders are frequently administered with meals in dialysis patients and often these will supplement dietary calcium intake so that the daily requirement is met (5). In patients with well-controlled phosphorus levels but with low calcium levels, extra supplementation of calcium between meals or at night may be warranted (96). In CKD (predialysis and dialysis) patients, calcium supplementation should be individualized based on calcium, phosphorus, and PTH laboratory values and the use of supplemental activated vitamin D.

CKD (predialysis and dialysis) patients who are receiving calcium-containing phosphate binders are at potential risk of hypercalcemia, especially when vitamin D, which increases intestinal absorption of calcium, is also prescribed (5,15,19,20,26,28,85,95,97). Hypercalcemia can lead to calcification in extraskeletal tissues such as the kidneys, lungs, eyes, joints, skin, and heart, resulting in complications such as deterioration of kidney function, impaired gas exchange in the lungs, and cardiovascular disease (2,15,22,79). Occurrence of cardiovascular calcification has also been directly linked to the level of calcium intake and is promoted by an elevated Ca x P level (22–24,77,79,98,99). The recommended levels for calcium and Ca x P product are currently being reevaluated based on the potential for metastatic calcification. In CKD (predialysis and dialysis) patients, it has been recommended to maintain total calcium levels between 9.2 and 9.6 mg/dL and a Ca x P product less than 50 to 55 (16,19,83). The calcium that is measured in the blood is the portion that is protein-bound. In situations where albumin levels are depressed, serum calcium levels may be artificially low. See Section 8 for further discussion on adjusting calcium levels for albumin levels.

If calcium levels or the Ca x P product become elevated, use of calcium-based binders, activated vitamin D use, and dialysate calcium levels should be reevaluated and adjusted (17,100). Several new therapies are available to help reduce the occurrence of hypercalcemia while still allowing for the prevention or treatment of hyperphosphatemia and hyperparathyroidism. Non-calcemic vitamin D analogs that can suppress PTH while having less impact on absorption of calcium in the intestine are now available (16,19,28). Calcium-free and aluminum-free phosphate binders are also now on the market, and can be used with or in place of calcium-based binders to reduce phosphorus levels without aggravating calcium or Ca x P levels (16,19,20,86,101). Recently, agents that activate the calcium-sensing receptor in the parathyroid gland have been developed (28,97,102). These agents, called calcimimetics, work independent of calcium and make the calcium-sensing receptor more sensitive to the suppressive effect of calcium on PTH secretion (102). This results in a decrease in PTH levels with a simlutaneous reduction in phosphorus and Ca x P levels and a small decrease in calcium levels (97,102).

Renal osteodystrophy is common in renal transplant patients. Immunosuppressive therapy, especially corticosteroids, can directly affect calcium metabolism and bone turnover (2,5). Calcium intake of 800 to 1,500 mg/day is recommended, with an increase in fluid intake to prevent formation of renal calcium stones (5,103). Bone status should be carefully monitored in transplant patients through the use of serum and urine calcium levels, PTH levels, and bone densitometry studies (5).

Magnesium

Because the kidney is the main route for excretion of magnesium, it plays a major role in magnesium regulation (88,104,105). As renal function declines, the kidney increases the fractional excretion of magnesium to maintain normal serum magnesium levels (104,105). When GFR drops below 10 to 15 mL/min, the compensatory increase in the fractional excretion is often no longer sufficient, and serum magnesium levels may begin to rise (5,104). Serum magnesium levels in dialysis patients are usually normal or slightly elevated, and hypermagnesemia, when it occurs, usually is mild and asymptomatic unless the patient takes medicines that contain large quantities of magnesium, such as magnesium-containing antacids and laxatives (5,104–108). In hemodialysis and peritoneal dialysis patients, serum magnesium levels are largely affected by the level of magnesium in the dialysate (2,104,105). An increased serum level of magnesium may suppress PTH, but it can also have a direct effect on bone histology and play a significant role in development of renal bone disease (5,105).

Magnesium salts, such as magnesium hydroxide and magnesium carbonate, have been used as phosphate binders with mixed results (109,110). Magnesium hydroxide resulted in poor phosphorus control in two different studies (110). Control of phosphorus seems to be effective with magnesium carbonate, but the large doses of magnesium required often lead to side effects such as diarrhea and hypermagnesemia (109,110). With the use of magnesium binders, dialysate magnesium levels need to be reduced to help avoid magnesium toxicity (28,109,110). Using a very low magnesium dialysate, however, could potentially lower serum magnesium levels drastically and pose a risk for cardiac arrhythmia or seizures (28).

Hypomagnesemia is rare in renal disease, although depressed levels may occur with the use of certain medications (eg, loop and thiazide diuretics, antibiotics, cisplatin, and cyclosporine) and in situations of acute alcohol intake, phosphate depletion, hypercalcemia, hyperparathyroidism, renal transplantation, acute pancreatitis, and the diuretic phase of acute renal failure (2,5,88,91). Low serum magnesium levels can interfere with the release of PTH and lead to hypocalcemia (5,88,93,104).

For CKD (predialysis and dialysis) patients, supplementation of magnesium is not recommended unless a magnesium deficiency is diagnosed. Magnesium intake should be limited in acute renal failure, with levels adjusted according to the clinical status of the patient (5). The recommended amount of magnesium to provide via TPN in acute renal failure is 4 mmol/day (5). Transplant recipients may experience hypomagnesemia with use of cyclosporin (5,88). Routine monitoring of magnesium levels in transplant recipients is suggested and supplementation with magnesium may be indicated (5).

Trace Minerals

Patients with CKD experience alterations in trace mineral metabolism; serum and/or tissue levels can be high or low. Trace minerals should be supplemented or restricted only after appropriate biochemical assessments.

Aluminum

Aluminum toxicity in dialysis patients has been a major concern in the past. Several factors can contribute to aluminum toxicity, including (90,111–115):

- Loss of the renal excretory pathway for aluminum
- Increased aluminum absorption from the gut due to uremia
- High aluminum concentrations in drinking water (and water used for dialysate if not properly purified)
- Aluminum in food and drinks
- Large amounts of aluminum-based phosphate binders (especially if administered with citrate compounds, see below)
- Albumin, hyperalimentation solutions (may contain substantial amounts of aluminum)

- Drugs containing aluminum (eg, antacids and buffered aspirin)
- Contaminated dialysis solutions

Other factors may increase the susceptibility to aluminum accumulation (111,114–119):

- Iron deficiency (increased intestinal absorption and possibly other mechanisms)
- Ingestion of substances facilitating aluminum absorption (eg, citrate and ascorbate, discussed later in this section)
- Diabetes (increased rate of whole-body aluminum accumulation)
- Hypoparathyroidism/parathyroidectomy
- Inflammatory bowel disease or short-bowel syndrome
- Steroid therapy

The prevalence of aluminum-related diseases in dialysis patients has diminished greatly in recent years due to the successful purification of the water used to prepare dialysate and the limited use of aluminum-based phosphate binders (114,116). The threat of aluminum toxicity has not been completely eradicated, however. A few patients do continue to use aluminum-based phosphate binders because they are not able to achieve a satisfactory control of serum phosphorus without their use (120,121).

Citrate (from sources such as Shohl's solution, calcium citrate, citrus fruit juices, and Alka-Seltzer) substantially enhances aluminum absorption, both by increasing aluminum solubility at neutral pH values and by augmenting paracellular intestinal permeability, and thus the concomitant use of citrate products and aluminum compounds should be avoided (2,5,90,111,113–115,122–125). For CKD (predialysis and dialysis) patients, in whom the potential for aluminum accumulation is increased, it has been suggested that even the use of soft drinks containing citrates be avoided because of the possibility of facilitated aluminum absorption (5,115). Ascorbate has also been shown to increase aluminum absorption, and it has been suggested that ascorbic acid supplementation, at least in large doses ($\geq$ 2 g/day), be avoided by CKD (predialysis and dialysis) patients who are ingesting aluminum preparations (5).

Aluminum toxicity in uremic patients is associated with several clinical problems including encephalopathy, dementia, vitamin D–resistant osteomalacia, adynamic bone disease, and microcytic anemia with resistance to EPO (2,5,90,111–113,116,120,126). An increased susceptibility to infections has also been noted (112,114,116,127).

Serum aluminum levels should be tested regularly in dialysis patients to detect any increase in exposure to aluminum and assess the risk for toxicity (2,115). In dialysis patients, aluminum levels less than 10 µg/L are considered desirable (2). Aluminum levels are highly associated with the development of aluminum-related bone disease, and patients with aluminum levels below 30 to 40 µg/L seem to be at lower risk, although development of aluminum-related bone disease is still possible (2,111,128). The risk of bone disease is much greater with serum aluminum levels more than 60 µg/L (111,115). In patients with severely increased aluminum levels, the use of deferoxamine (DFO), a chelating agent, has been used to remove aluminum (5,90,111,115,129). However, DFO treatment may have serious side effects and much caution should be exercised if it is used (90,111,119,129,130). Reported side effects of DFO include vision impairment, retinopathy, ototoxicity, hypotension, depletion of iron stores, bacterial and fungal infections, and neurotoxicity (5,90,111,119,129,130). Overzealous use of DFO may induce enhanced aluminum toxicity by itself as well (5,111). It is preferable to first attempt to treat increased aluminum levels by identifying and eliminating all possible contributors to the aluminum accumulation. With the advent of noncalcium-based, non–aluminum-based phosphate binders, it may be possible to eliminate the need for the use of aluminum-based phosphate binders in renal patients.

Iron

Iron deficiency is common in CKD (predialysis and dialysis) patients, particularly patients on hemodialysis, and is primarily due to the substantial losses of blood from frequent blood tests, blood remaining in the dialysis tubing and dialyzer, and gastrointestinal blood losses (131–135). Iron availability may also be limited because of increased gastric pH from phosphate binder use, aluminum ingestion or overload, or hyperparathyroidism (132,136,137). Also, it has been suggested that the absorption of iron in uremic patients may be additionally compromised, possibly due in part to inflammatory processes (133,135,137,138). In patients receiving recombinant human erythropoietin (EPO), the need for iron is compounded because of the increased rate of erythropoiesis (5,131,134).

The measures commonly used to assess iron status in CKD patients are serum ferritin and transferrin saturation (131,134,136,138,139). To ensure adequate iron availability, serum ferritin should be maintained at 100 ng/mL or more and transferrin saturation at 20% or more (131,134). Low ferritin levels (< 100 ng/mL) indicate absolute iron deficiency, in which iron stores are depleted and negative iron balance ensues (131,136,138–140). High ferritin levels, however, do not exclude functional iron deficiency, a condition in which iron stores are adequate but iron release from the stores is impaired or inadequate (131,135,136,138,139). The use of EPO can stimulate erythropoiesis to such an extent that the demand for iron can exceed the body's ability to release it from stores (139,140). Functional iron deficiency is defined by normal or high ferritin levels, but transferrin saturation less than 20% (131,136,138–140). Both absolute and functional iron deficiency are indications that iron therapy may be warranted (138,139).

Two newer methods for determining iron needs are also available but are not widely used in the United States. The percentage of hypochromic red blood cells (red cells with a cell hemoglobin concentration < 28 g/dL) reflects the adequacy of the iron supply (135,141). When the percentage of hypochromic red blood cells is more than 10%, iron deficiency is strongly suggested and iron supplementation should be considered (131,135,140–143). Reticulocyte hemoglobin content is another method for detecting iron deficiency. The hemoglobin content of reticulocytes is more stable than serum ferritin and transferrin saturation and will decrease when iron deficiency is present (140,141). Levels less than 29 pg are indicative of iron deficiency and the need for iron supplementation (141,142).

Many patients receiving regular EPO therapy will require oral or intravenous iron supplementation (131,134,138). Often, oral iron supplementation is the first route used and may be sufficient for CKD (predialysis) and peritoneal dialysis patients (131,135,140,143,144). Supplemental elemental iron in doses of 150 to 200 mg/day for CKD (predialysis) patients and 200 mg/day for peritoneal dialysis patients has been suggested (131,140). The absorption of iron in the gut is not efficient, however, and may be impaired by several factors. To maximize absorption, the supplements should be taken more than 2 hours after or more than 1 hour before meals and should not be taken with binders (131). Oral vitamin C may help increase absorption of iron, but supplementation with more than 100 mg/day of vitamin C is contraindicated in CKD patients due to the risk of oxalosis (133). Side effects from oral iron are common, including constipation, nausea, heartburn, bloating, diarrhea, altered taste, and abdominal cramps, and these adverse effects may affect patient compliance (5,133,136). Sustained-release tablets reduce these effects, but may not be as effective because they disintegrate farther down the GI tract than the duodenum and proximal jejunum where iron is maximally absorbed (133,136). If CKD (predialysis) and peritoneal dialysis patients are unable to maintain adequate iron status with oral iron, use of intravenous iron will become necessary (140). Because of the increased blood losses with the hemodialysis procedure, hemodialysis patients typically have difficulty keeping iron stores at adequate levels with oral iron and require intravenous iron supplementation (131,134,138,140).

Three forms of intravenous iron are available in the United States: iron dextran, iron gluconate, and iron sucrose. All three forms of iron are effective at repleting iron stores, but iron dextran has the potential for causing anaphylactic reactions in a small number of patients (140,143,145–147). Other side effects noted with the use of iron dextran include hypotension, nausea, vomiting, diarrhea, abdominal pain, headache, flushing, urticaria, pruritis, malaise, myalgia, fever, and leukocyte dysfunction (143,146,148). Adverse side effects, including hypotension, nausea, vomiting, diarrhea, flushing, epigastric pain, chest pain, and paresthesias have been reported with the use of iron gluconate (131,143,146). Reports of adverse effects with the use of iron sucrose are rare, with hypotension, back pain, vomiting, vertigo, flushing, and urticaria being some of the few documented (146). Recommendations for administration of intravenous iron in CKD patients have been established and are available in the NKF-K/DOQI Guidelines (131).

Iron overload may occur with the use of intravenous iron. Several consequences of iron overload have been suggested, such as insulin resistance, liver cirrhosis, cardiac dysfunction, increased generation of free radicals, and increased susceptibility to infections (5,131,132,138,139,145,149,150). Controversy exists, though, about whether many of these consequences are a result of iron overload. There is no consensus about the recommended levels for determining iron overload. Suggested levels range from 500 to 1,000 ng/mL for ferritin, with transferrin saturation levels generally set at 50% or more (131,135,138,139,151,152). Elevated ferritin levels are not specific for iron overload, however, because ferritin can be elevated in response to inflammatory and infectious processes (133,136,139,152). It has been proposed that, to avoid excessive iron accumulation, intravenous iron supplementation should be held for up to 3 months in patients in whom transferrin saturation is 50% or more and/or serum ferritin is 800 ng/mL or more (131,134,152).

The use of intravenous vitamin C has been proposed as a method to improve hematologic indexes in patients with high ferritin levels who are resistant to EPO (135,153). Concerns have been expressed about the use of this therapy and the risk of oxalosis. Few studies, however, have looked at oxalate levels with the infusion of vitamin C. In one study on intravenous vitamin C use in hemodialysis patients, only 50% of the patients responded to intravenous vitamin C therapy, and in those who responded the effect of the therapy seemed to only last the duration of the treatment (152,153). Oxalate levels increased steadily over the duration of the study in both responders and nonresponders, although not significantly (152,153). The study only lasted 8 weeks, however, and it is not clear whether oxalate levels would continue to increase and reach a significant level with longer duration of treatment (152). It has been suggested that use of intravenous vitamin C be limited until further studies investigating the risks associated with this treatment be completed (152).

Iron status should be monitored regularly, especially in patients who are receiving EPO therapy. In patients receiving EPO but not receiving intravenous iron, iron status should be monitored monthly during the initiation of therapy and then at least once every 3 months after the target hemoglobin level is attained (131). Patients receiving intravenous iron and EPO should have iron status checked at least once every 3 months, and those who have adequate iron levels and are not receiving EPO should have iron status checked every 3 to 6 months (131).

The most common cause of incomplete response to EPO therapy is iron deficiency (131,143,144). If an inadequate response to EPO exists despite adequate iron status, other possible causes should be evaluated and treated (131). Section 13 lists the possible causes for inadequate response to EPO.

Zinc

Zinc metabolism seems to be altered in patients with CKD, particularly those with nephrotic syndrome, CKD (predialysis), or renal transplants (2,154-156). There is controversy about the zinc status and its significance in CKD due to the lack of definitive criteria for diagnosis of zinc deficiency and the variability of zinc plasma and tissue levels (6,154). However, several factors that could lead to zinc deficiency are common in CKD patients. Low protein intake, malabsorption, anorexia, nausea, and vomiting, all common problems in CKD patients, can affect zinc status (154,156). Several medications that CKD patients commonly use interfere with zinc absorption, including calcium, iron, and phosphate binders (5,154,156). Penicillamine and corticosteroids have also been associated with zinc deficiency (5,154,156). Patients on hemodialysis may also have increased fecal zinc excretion, which may be a major contributor to negative zinc balance (155,156). Hypozincemia can persist despite renal transplantation, due to a marked increase in urinary zinc excretion possibly from the use of immunosuppressive drugs (5,154,157,158).

Growth retardation, delayed wound healing, decreased taste acuity, impotence, glucose intolerance, hyperlipidemia, skin changes, mental lethargy, anemia, and reduced resistance to infections are all characteristics of zinc deficiency (2,154,156,157). Improvements in taste, smell, appetite, wound healing, immune function, anemia, and sexual function have been reported in CKD patients supplemented with zinc (2,5,156,159), but the results have not been confirmed (2).

Because of the lack of concrete information about the benefits of zinc supplementation, the current recommendation is that supplements not be routinely prescribed as long as CKD (predialysis and dialysis) patients maintain an intake of zinc at or above the DRI (8–11 mg/day) (5). However, zinc supplementation for transplant recipients in the amount of 15 mg/day has been suggested (2,5). In patients with complaints of a poor appetite, lack of energy, skin changes, taste abnormalities, weight loss, recurring infections, difficulty with wound healing, or gonadal dysfunction, zinc supplementation may be beneficial (5,6,156,159). For these patients, 50 mg/day of elemental zinc is a fairly common dose, although an optimal level of supplementation has not been determined (156). Oral supplements of zinc sulfate and zinc gluconate are available and can be obtained over-the-counter. Because of the interaction between iron and both calcium-based and aluminum-based phosphate binders, zinc should not be taken at the same time as these medications (156,160). Zinc absorption is also reduced by phytic acid, fiber, and alcohol (161). Zinc supplementation, even as little as 25 mg/day, can reduce copper status and excess zinc can lead to a copper deficiency, so patients taking zinc supplements may need to be monitored for hypocupremia (156,160-163).

Monitoring of zinc status by plasma levels may not be reliable (2,6,156,160). Low plasma zinc levels can be suggestive of deficiency but are not diagnostic (154). Also, plasma zinc levels can vary in situations of stress, including renal failure (2). In dialysis patients, plasma zinc levels are often low, but red blood cell zinc is typically normal or elevated (5,154,164,165). Additionally, a majority of zinc in the plasma is bound to albumin, so plasma zinc levels may be artificially low when albumin levels are decreased (2,162). Routine monitoring of patients receiving zinc supplementation can be accomplished through other methods, such as assessment of clinical response through improvement of symptoms or by functional tests (154,156).

Selenium

Selenium is an essential trace mineral important for glutathione peroxidase (GPX), an enzyme that protects cells from lipid peroxidation (2,162). Low plasma selenium levels and GPX levels have been reported in CKD (predialysis and dialysis) patients (5,150,166–170). It has also been found that the kidney is the main source of the plasma or extracellular form of GPX, and that extracellular GPX is reduced by 42% in hemodialysis patients (166,169). Serum selenium concentrations and GPX activity are typically used to evaluate selenium status (166,167).

Deficiency of selenium has been linked to cardiomyopathy, skeletal myopathy, increased risks of cardiovascular disease and cancer, anemia, and immune dysfunction, all of which are frequently associated with chronic uremia resulting from renal disease (5,166,167). A few investigators have studied the effectiveness of selenium supplementation in hemodialysis patients. An increase in GPX activity and an improvement in immune parameters have been reported by some, whereas others have shown no improvement in GPX activity with supplementation of selenium (166,168–170). Currently, there is no standard recommendation for supplementation of selenium in CKD patients. Retention of selenium in CKD patients could be a concern because selenium homeostasis is maintained primarily through urinary excretion (166). Supplementation, if provided, should thus be monitored closely (166). Physical symptoms of selenium toxicity include hair and nail changes, nausea and vomiting, garlic or sour milk breath odor, peripheral neuropathy, and fatigue (150,161,166,171).

Copper

Serum copper levels are usually normal in CKD (predialysis and dialysis) patients, although levels in dialysis patients have been reported to be lower than those of control subjects (6,106,150,164,165,172). Copper deficiency is not commonly seen in uremia, except perhaps in the cases of severely ill patients with prolonged hospitalizations (5). A decrease in blood copper may occur in nephrotic syndrome due to the increased urinary loss of ceruloplasmin-bound copper, but this does not cause clinically recognized manifestations (2,5,150).

Zinc interferes with copper absorption, and therapeutic levels of zinc supplementation can lead to copper deficiency (160–162,173). High intakes of iron, ascorbic acid, or fructose also seem to decrease copper bioavailability (161,162,173). Copper deficiency has been associated with ischemic heart disease (5).

Oral supplements of copper sulfate are typically given to treat copper deficiency in non-CKD patients with functional GI tracts (161). Doses of as much as 2 mg/day are generally adequate to reverse the deficiency (161). No information is available regarding a safe dose for CKD patients.

Copper excess has been linked to lipid oxidation, accelerated atherogenesis, and excess risk of myocardial infarction, and can result in liver cirrhosis (5, 161). Initial signs of copper toxicity include metallic taste, nausea, vomiting, epigastric pain, headache diarrhea, hemolysis, and hyperglycemia (150). Anuria, hypotension, and coma occur in the most severe cases (150).

Chromium

Chromium levels tend to increase with chronic dialysis treatment (5,150,157,174). The cause of these elevated levels may be the result of chromium exposure during dialysis (157,174).

Chromium plays an important role in carbohydrate and lipid metabolism as the metal component and activator in glucose tolerance factor, and is required for optimal utilization of glucose (150,160–162).

There are no simple tests to assess chromium status (161). The only reliable approach is to monitor glucose and lipid levels before and after chromium supplementation, and if chromium was deficient, serum glucose or lipid levels should return to normal (161). Because chromium is an essential nutrient, further research is needed to investigate the effects of abnormally high serum chromium values in dialysis patients. There are no reports of chromium toxicity from dietary chromium, but toxicity has been documented from ingestion of contaminated drinking water and inhalation of chromium from industrial pollutants (161). Due to potential toxic effects, supplementation is not recommended.

Silicon

Plasma silicon levels are elevated in dialysis patients (5,150,175). This increase has been attributed to excess silicon concentration in the dialysate, as well as consumption of drinking water containing silicon (5,175). No overt effects of silicon accumulation have been noted with these increased levels (175).

References

1. Muth I. Implications of hypervitaminosis A in chronic renal failure. *J Ren Nutr*. 1991;1:2–8.

2. Mitch WE, Klahr S, eds. *Handbook of Nutrition and the Kidney*. 3rd ed. Philadelphia, Pa: Lippincott-Raven Publishers, 1998.

3. Chen J, He J, Odgen LG, Batuman V, Whelton PK. Relationship of serum antioxidant vitamins to serum creatinine in the US population. *Am J Kidney Dis*. 2002;39:460–468.

4. Jahnke MG, Rock CL, Carter CM, Kelly MP, Gorenfo DW, Messana JM, Swartz RD, Rehan A, Jones MF, Lipschutz D. Antioxidant vitamins and carotenoids in hemodialysis and peritoneal dialysis patients. *J Ren Nutr*. 1996;6:79–88.

5. Kopple JD, Massry SG, eds. *Nutritional Management of Renal Disease*. Baltimore, Md: Williams & Wilkins; 1997.

6. Wolk R. Micronutrition in dialysis. *Nutr Clin Pract*. 1993;8:267–276.

7. Audran M, Gross M, Kumar R. The physiology of the vitamin D endocrine system. *Semin Nephrol*. 1986;6:4–20.

8. Malluche HH, Mawad H, Koszewski NJ. Update on vitamin D and its newer analogues: actions and rationale for treatment in chronic renal failure. *Kidney Int*. 2002;62:367–374.

9. Dusso AS, Brown AJ. Mechanism of vitamin D action and its regulation. *Am J Kidney Dis.* 1998;32(4 Suppl 2):S13–S24.

10. McCarthy JT, Kumar R. Behavior of the vitamin D endocrine system in the development of renal osteodystrophy. *Semin Nephrol.* 1986;6:21–30.

11. National Kidney Foundation Kidney Disease Outcome Quality Initiative Advisory Board. K/DOQI clinical practice guidelines for chronic kidney disease: evaluation, classification, and stratification. *Am J Kidney Dis.* 2002;39(2 Suppl 2):S1–S246.

12. Lu KC, Lin SH, Chyr SH, Shieh SD. Influence of metabolic acidosis on serum $1,25(OH)_2D_3$ levels in chronic renal failure. *Miner Electrolyte Metab.* 1995;21:398–402.

13. Slatopolsky E, Dusso A, Brown AJ. Control of uremic bone disease: role of vitamin D analogs. *Kidney Int.* 2002;61(Suppl 80):S143–S148.

14. Fukagawa M, Kitaoka M, Kurokawa K. Resistance of the parathyroid glands to vitamin D in renal failure: implications for medical management. *Kidney Int.* 1997;52(Suppl 62):S60–S64.

15. Slatopolsky E, Brown A, Dusso A. Role of phosphorus in the pathogenesis of secondary hyperparathyroidism. *Am J Kidney Dis.* 2001;37(1 Suppl 2):S54–S57.

16. Malluche HH, Monier-Faugere MC. Understanding and managing hyperphosphatemia in patients with chronic renal disease. *Clin Nephrol.* 1999;52:267–277.

17. Leavey SF, Weitzel WF. Endocrine abnormalities in chronic renal failure. *Endocrinol Metab Clin North Am.* 2002;31:107–119.

18. Llach F, Yudd M. The importance of hyperphosphataemia in the severity of hyperparathyroidism and its treatment in patients with chronic renal failure. *Nephrol Dial Transplant.* 1998;13(Suppl 3):57–61.

19. Block GA, Port FK. Re-evaluation of risks associated with hyperphosphatemia and hyperparathyroidism in dialysis patients: recommendations for a change in management. *Am J Kidney Dis.* 2000;35:1226–1237.

20. Bleyer AJ, Burke SK, Dillon M, Garrett B, Kant KS, Lynch D, Rahman SN, Schoenfeld P, Teitelbaum I, Zeig S, Slatopolsky E. A comparison of the calcium-free phosphate binder sevelamer hydrochloride with calcium acetate in the treatment of hyperphosphatemia in hemodialysis patients. *Am J Kidney Dis.* 1999;33:694–701.

21. Rostand SG, Drüeke TB. Parathyroid hormone, vitamin D, and cardiovascular disease in chronic renal failure. *Kidney Int.* 1999;56:383–392.

22. Llach F. Cardiac calcification: dealing with another risk factor in patients with kidney failure. *Semin Dial.* 1999;12:293–295.

23. Ribeiro S, Ramos A, Brandão A, Rebelo JR, Guerra A, Resina C, Vila-Lobos A, Carvalho F, Remédio F, Ribeiro F. Cardiac valve calcification in haemodialysis patients: role of calcium-phosphate metabolism. *Nephrol Dial Transplant.* 1998;13:2037–2040.

24. Ahmed S, O'Neill KD, Hood AF, Evan AP, Moe SM. Calciphylaxis is associated with hyperphosphatemia and increased osteopontin expression by vascular smooth muscle cells. *Am J Kidney Dis.* 2001;37:1267–1276.

25. Drüeke TB. Control of secondary hyperparathyroidism by vitamin D derivatives. *Am J Kidney Dis.* 2001;37(1 Suppl 2):S58–S61.

26. Tsuchihashi K, Takizawa H, Torii TA, Ikeda R, Nakahara N, Yuda S, Kobayashi N, Nakata T, Nobuyuki U, Shimamoto K. Hypoparathyroidism potentiates cardiovascular complications through disturbed calcium metabolism: possible risk of vitamin D_3 analog administration in dialysis patients with end-stage renal disease. *Nephron.* 2000;84:13–20.

27. Jernigan P, Andress DL. Vitamin D analogs in uremia: integrating medical and nutritional issues. *J Ren Nutr.* 2001;11:3–8.

28. Chertow GM, Martin KJ. Current and future therapies for the medical management of secondary hyperparathyroidism. *Semin Dial.* 1998;11:267–270.

29. Caravaca F, Fernández MA, Cubero J, Aparicio A, Jimenez F, García MC. Are plasma 1,25-dihyroxyvitamin D_3 concentrations appropriate after successful kidney transplantation? *Nephrol Dial Transplant.* 1998;13(Suppl 3):91–93.

30. Gentile MG, Porrini M, Manna GM, Ciceri R, Cofano F, Simonetti P, D'Amico G. Water- and fat-soluble vitamin status in chronic renal insufficiency patients. *Contrib Nephrol.* 1992;98:89–97.

31. Roca AO, Jarjoura D, Blend D, Cugino A, Rutecki GW, Nuchikat PS, Whittier FC. Dialysis leg cramps: efficacy of quinine versus vitamin D. *ASAIO J*. 1992;38:M481–M485.

32. Khajehdehi P, Mojerlou M, Behzadi S, Rais-Jalali GA. A randomized, double-blind, placebo-controlled trial of supplementary vitamins E, C and their combination for treatment of haemodialysis cramps. *Nephrol Dial Transplant*. 2001;16:1448–1451.

33. Clermont G, Lecour S, Cabanne JF, Motte G, Guilland JC, Chevet D, Rochette L. Vitamin D-coated dialyzer reduces oxidative stress in hemodialysis patients. *Free Radic Biol Med*. 2001;31:233–241.

34. Satoh M, Yamasaki Y, Nagake Y, Kasahara J, Hashimoto M, Nakanishi N, Makino H. Oxidative stress is reduced by the long-term use of vitamin E-coated dialysis filters. *Kidney Int*. 2001;59:1943–1950.

35. Kohlmeier M, Saupe J, Shearer MJ, Schaefer K, Asmus G. Bone health of adult hemodialysis patients is related to vitamin K status. *Kidney Int*. 1997;51:1218–1221.

36. Makoff R. Vitamin supplementation in persons with renal disease. *EDTNA ERCA J*. 1992;18:11–14.

37. Makoff R. The risk of oxalosis in patients with renal disease. *Nephrology Forum*. 1992;1:1,4.

38. Shah GM, Ross EA, Sabo A, Pichon M, Reynolds RD, Bhagavan H. Effects of ascorbic acid and pyridoxine supplementation on oxalate metabolism in peritoneal dialysis patients. *Am J Kidney Dis*. 1992;20:42–49.

39. Alkhunaizi AM, Chan L. Secondary oxalosis: a cause of delayed recovery of renal function in the setting of acute renal failure. *J Am Soc Nephrol*. 1996;7:2320–2326.

40. Ono K. Secondary hyperoxalemia caused by vitamin C supplementation in regular hemodialysis patients. *Clin Nephrol*. 1986;25:239–243.

41. Rolton HA, McConnell KM, Modi KS, MacDougall AI. The effect of vitamin C intake on plasma oxalate in patients on regular hemodialysis. *Nephol Dial Transplant*. 1991;6:440–443.

42. Descombes E, Hanck AB, Fellay G. Water-soluble vitamins in chronic hemodialysis patients and need for supplementation. *Kidney Int*. 1993;43:1319–1328.

43. Tamura T, Johnston KE, Bergman SM. Homocysteine and folate concentrations in blood from patients treated with hemodialysis. *J Am Soc Nephrol*. 1996;7:2414–2418.

44. Robinson K, Gupta A, Dennis V, Arheart K, Chaudhary D, Green R, Vigo P, Mayer E, Selhub J, Kutner M, Jacobsen DW. Hyperhomocysteinemia confers an independent increased risk of atherosclerosis in end-stage renal disease and is closely linked to plasma folate and pyridoxine concentrations. *Circulation*. 1996;94:2743–2748.

45. Dennis V, Robinson K. Homocysteinemia and vascular disease in end-stage renal disease. *Kidney Int*. 1996;50(Suppl 57):S11-S17.

46. Leblanc M, Pichette V, Geadah D, Ouimet D. Folic acid and pyridoxal-5'-phosphate losses during high-efficiency hemodialysis in patients without hydrosoluble vitamin supplementation. *J Ren Nutr*. 2000;10:196–201.

47. Arnadottir M, Brattström L, Simonsen O, Thysell H, Hultburg B, Andersson A, Nilsson-Ehle P. The effect of high-dose pyridoxine and folic acid supplementation on serum lipid and plasma homocysteine concentrations in dialysis patients. *Clin Nephrol*. 1993;40:236–240.

48. Clarke R, Armitage J. Vitamin supplements and cardiovascular risk: review of the randomized trials of homocysteine-lowering vitamin supplements. *Semin Thromb Hemost*. 2000;26:341–348.

49. Naruszewicz M, Klinke M, Dziewanowski K, Staniewicz A, Bukowska H. Homocysteine, fibrinogen, and lipoprotein(a) levels are simultaneously reduced in patients with chronic renal failure treated with folic acid, pyridoxine, and cyanocobalamin. *Metabolism*. 2001;50:131–134.

50. Billion S, Tribout B, Cadet E, Queinnec C, Rochette J, Wheatley P, Bataille P. Hyperhomocysteinaemia, folate and vitamin B-12 in unsupplemented haemodialysis patients: effect of oral therapy with folic acid and vitamin B-12. *Nephrol Dial Transplant*. 2002;17:455–461.

51. Chauveau P, Chadefaux B, Coudé M, Aupetit J, Kamoun P, Jungers P. Long-term folic acid (but not pyridoxine) supplementation lowers elevated plasma homocysteine level in chronic renal failure. *Miner Electrolyte Metab*. 1996;22:106–109.

52. Jannssen MJFM, van Guldener C, de Jong GMT, van den Berg M, Stehouwer CDA, Donker AJM. Folic acid treatment of hyperhomocysteinemia in dialysis patients. *Miner Electrolyte Metab*. 1996;22:110–114.

53. Bostom AG, Lathrop L. Hyperhomocysteinemia in end-stage renal disease: prevalence, etiology, and potential relationship to arteriosclerotic outcomes. *Kidney Int.* 1997;52:10–20.

54. Van Guldener C, Robinson K. Homocysteine and renal disease. *Semin Thromb Hemost.* 2000;26:313–324.

55. Dierkes J, Domröse U, Bosselmann KP, Neumann KH, Luley C. Homocysteine-lowering effect of different multivitamin preparations in patients with end-stage renal disease. *J Ren Nutr.* 2001;11:67–72.

56. Bostom AG, Shemin D, Gohh RY, Beaulieu AJ, Jacques PF, Dworkin L, Selhub J. Treatment of mild hyperhomocysteinemia in renal transplant recipients versus hemodialysis patients. *Transplantation.* 2000;69:2128–2131.

57. Beaulieu AJ, Gohh RY, Han H, Hakas D, Jacques PF, Selhub J, Bostom AG. Enhanced reduction of fasting total homocysteine levels with supraphysiological versus standard multivitamin dose folic acid supplementation in renal transplant recipients. *Arterioscler Thromb Vasc Biol.*1999;19:2918–2921.

58. Stanford JL, Molina H, Phillips J, Kohlman-Trigoboff D, Moore J, Smith BM. Oral folate reduces plasma homocysteine levels in hemodialysis patients with cardiovascular disease. *Cardiovasc Surg.* 2000;8:567–571.

59. Manns B, Hyndman E, Burgess E, Parsons H, Schaefer J, Snyder F, Scott-Douglas N. Oral vitamin B-12 and high-dose folic acid in hemodialysis patients with hyperhomocysteinemia. *Kidney Int.* 2001;59:1103–1109.

60. McGregor D, Shand B, Lynn K. A controlled trial of the effect of folate supplements on homocysteine, lipids, and hemorheology in end-stage renal disease. *Nephron.* 2000;85:215–220.

61. Grandtnerová B, Laca L, Gábor D, Gregová E, Korónyi S. Folic acid supplements and homocysteine level in renal transplant recipients. *Transplant Proceed.* 2001;33:2049–2050.

62. De Vecchi AF, Patrosso C, Novembrino C, Finazzi S, Colucci P, De Franceschi M, Fasano MA, Bamonti-Catena F. Folate supplementation in peritoneal dialysis patients with normal erythrocyte folate: effect on plasma homocysteine. *Nephron.* 2001;89:297–302.

63. Beto JA, Bansal VK. Interventions for other risk factors: tobacco use, physical inactivity, menopause, and homocysteine. *Am J Kidney Dis.* 1998;32(5, Suppl 3):S172–S184.

64. Makoff R, Dwyer J, Rocco MV. Folic acid, pyridoxine, cobalamin, and homocysteine and their relationship to cardiovascular disease in end-stage renal disease. *J Ren Nutr.* 1996;6:2–11.

65. Bostom AG, Lathrop L. Hyperhomocysteinemia in end-stage renal disease: prevalence, etiology, and potential relationship to arteriosclerotic outcomes. *Kidney Int.* 1997;52:10–20.

66. Rock CL, Bidigare DeRoeck M, Gorenflo DW, Jahnke MG, Swartz RD, Messana JM. Current prevalence of vitamin B-6 deficiency in hemodialysis and peritoneal dialysis patients. *J Ren Nutr.* 1997;7:10–16.

67. Laso Guzmán FJ, González-Buitrago JM, Vela R, Cava F, de Castro S. Vitamin B6 status in uremia. *Klin Wochenschr.* 1990;68:183–186.

68. Lindner A, Bankson DD, Stehman-Breen C, Mahuren JD, Coburn SP. Vitamin B6 metabolism and homocysteine in end-stage renal disease and chronic renal insufficiency. *Am J Kidney Dis.* 2002;39:134–145.

69. Tamura T, Bergman SM, Morgan SL. Homocysteine, B vitamins, and vascular-access thrombosis in patients treated with hemodialysis. *Am J Kidney Dis.* 1998;32:475–481.

70. Mydlík M, Derzsiová K, Zemberová E. Metabolism of vitamin B6 and its requirement in chronic renal failure. *Kidney Int.* 1997;52(Suppl 62):S56–S59.

71. Bostom AG, Shemin D, Gohh RY, Beaulieu AJ, Bagley P, Massy ZA, Jacques PF, Dworkin L, Selhub J. Treatment of hyperhomocysteinemia in hemodialysis patients and renal transplant recipients. *Kidney Int.* 2001;59(Suppl 78):S246–S252.

72. Zeman FJ. *Clinical Nutrition and Dietetics.* 2nd ed. New York, NY: Macmillan Publishing; 1991.

73. Mahan LK, Escott-Stump S, eds. *Krause's Food Nutrition, and Diet Therapy.* 10th ed. Philadelphia, Pa: WB Saunders; 2000.

74. Schneede J, Refsum H, Ueland PM. Biological and environmental determinants of plasma homocysteine. *Semin Thromb Hemost.* 2000;26:263–279.

75. Elian KM, Hoffer LJ. Hydroxocobalamin reduces hyperhomocysteinemia in end-stage renal disease. *Metabolism.* 2002;51:881–886.

76. Llach F, Yudd M. Pathogenic, clinical, and therapeutic aspects of secondary hyperparathyroidism in chronic renal failure. *Am J Kidney Dis.* 1998;32(4 Suppl 2):S3–S12.

77. Delmez JA, Slatopolsky E. Hyperphosphatemia: its consequences and treatment in patients with chronic renal disease. *Am J Kidney Dis*. 1992;19:303–317.

78. Kates DM, Sherrard DJ, Andress DL. Evidence that serum phosphate is independently associated with serum PTH in patients with chronic renal failure. *Am J Kidney Dis*. 1997;30:809–813.

79. Norris KC. Toward a new treatment paradigm for hyperphosphatemia in chronic renal disease. *Dial Transplant*. 1998;27:767–773.

80. Marchais SJ, Metivier F, Guerin AP, London GM. Association of hyperphosphatemia with haemodynamic disturbances in end-stage renal disease. *Nephrol Dial Transplant*. 1999;14:2178–2183.

81. Block GA, Hulbert-Shearon TE, Levin NW, Port FK. Association of serum phosphorus and calcium x phosphate product with mortality risk in chronic hemodialysis patients: a national study. *Am J Kidney Dis*. 1998;31:607–617.

82. Amann K, Gross ML, London GM, Ritz E. Hyperphosphatemia—a silent killer of patients with renal failure? *Nephrol Dial Transplant*. 1999;14:2085–2087.

83. Cannata-Andia JB, Rodriquez-Garcia M. Hyperphosphatemia as a cardiovascular risk factor—how to manage the problem. *Nephrol Dial Transplant*. 2002;17(Suppl 11):16–19.

84. Coburn JW. Mineral metabolism and renal bone disease: effects of CAPD versus hemodialysis. *Kidney Int*. 1993;43(Suppl 40):S92–S100.

85. Hamdy NAT, Brown CB, Boletis J, Boyle G, Tindale W, Beneton MNC, Charlesworth D, Kanis JA. Mineral metabolism in CAPD. *Contrib Nephrol*. 1990;85:100–110.

86. McIntyre CW, Patel V, Taylor GS, Fluck RJ. A prospective study of combination therapy for hyperphosphatemia with calcium-containing phosphate binders and sevelamer in hypercalcaemic haemodialysis patients. *Nephrol Dial Transplant*. 2002;17:1643–1648.

87. Walls J, Bennett SE. Maintaining nutrition in CAPD patients. *Contrib Nephrol*. 1990;85:79–83.

88. Weisinger JR, Bellorín-Font E. Magnesium and phosphorus. *Lancet*. 1998;352:391–396.

89. Stamatakis MK, Alderman JM, Meyer-Stout PJ. Influence of pH on in vitro disintegration of phosphate binders. *Am J Kidney Dis*. 1998;32:808–812.

90. Stover J, ed. *A Clinical Guide to Nutrition Care in End-Stage Renal Disease*. 2nd ed. Chicago, Ill: American Dietetic Association; 1994.

91. Vamvakas S, Teschner M, Bahner U, Heidland A. Alcohol abuse: potential role in electrolyte disturbances and kidney diseases. *Clin Nephrol*. 1998;49:205–213.

92. Goldstein DJ, Abrahamian-Gebeshian C. Nutrition support in renal failure. In: Matarese LE, Gottschlich MM. *Contemporary Nutrition Support Practice: A Clinical Guide*. Philadelphia, Pa: WB Saunders; 1998:447–471.

93. Bourke E, Delaney V. Assessment of hypocalcemia and hypercalcemia. *Clin Lab Med*. 1993;13:157–181.

94. Winchester JF, Rotellar C, Goggins M, Robino D, Rakowski TA, Argy WP. Calcium and phosphate balance in dialysis patients. *Kidney Int*. 1993;43(Suppl 41):S174–S178.

95. Blumenkrantz MJ. Nutrition. In: Daugirdas JT, Ing TS, eds. *Handbook of Dialysis*. 2nd ed. Boston, Mass: Little Brown; 1994:374–400.

96. Delmez JA, Slatopolsky E. Recent advances in the pathogenesis and therapy of uremic secondary hyperparathyroidism. *J Clin Endocrinol Metab*. 1991;72:735–739.

97. Drüeke TB. Treatment of secondary hyperparathyroidism with vitamin D derivatives and calcimimetics before and after start of dialysis. *Nephrol Dial Transplant*. 2002;17(Suppl 11):20–22.

98. Guérin AP, London GM, Marchais SJ, Metivier F. Arterial stiffening and vascular calcifications in end-stage renal disease. *Nephrol Dial Transplant*. 2000;15:1014–1021.

99. Goodman WG, Goldin J, Kuizon BD, Yoon C, Gales B, Sider D, Wang Y, Chung J, Emerick A, Greaser L, Elashoff RM, Salusky IB. Coronary-artery calcification in young adults with end-stage renal disease who are undergoing dialysis. *N Engl J Med*. 2000;342:1478–1483.

100. Korkor A, Blanchard M. Renal osteodystrophy management with CQI techniques. *Nephrology Exchange*. 1996;6:10–15.

101. Chertow GM, Burke SK, Dillon MA, Slatopolsky E. Long-term effects of sevelamer hydrochloride on the calcium x phosphate product and lipid profile of haemodialysis patients. *Nephrol Dial Transplant*. 1999;14:2907–2914.

102. Frazão JM, Martins P, Coburn JW. The calcimimetic agents: perspectives for treatment. *Kidney Int.* 2002;61(Suppl 80):S149–S154.

103. Pagenkemper JJ, Foulks CJ. Nutritional management of the adult renal transplant patient. *J Ren Nutr* 1991;1:119–124.

104. Mountokalakis TD. Magnesium metabolism in chronic renal failure. *Magnesium Res.* 1990;3:121–127.

105. Navarro-González JF. Magnesium in dialysis patients: serum levels and clinical implications. *Clin Nephrol.* 1998;49:373–378.

106. Krachler M, Scharfetter H, Wirnsberger GH. Kinetics of the metal cations magnesium, calcium, copper, zinc, strontium, barium, and lead in chronic hemodialysis patients. *Clin Nephrol.* 2000;54:35–44.

107. Pedrozzi NE, Truttmann AC, Faraone R, Descoeudres CE, Wermuth B, Lüthy CM, Nuoffer JM, Frey FJ, Bianchetti MG. Circulating ionized and total magnesium in end-stage kidney disease. *Nephron.* 1998;79:288–292.

108. Krachler M, Wirnsberger GH. Long-term changes of plasma trace element concentrations in chronic hemodialysis patients. *Blood Purif.* 2000;18:138–143.

109. Emmett M, Hootkins R. Phosphorus binders. *Nephrology Exchange.* 1992;2:7–12.

110. Malluche HH, Mawad H. Management of hyperphosphataemia of chronic kidney disease: lessons from the past and future directions. *Nephrol Dial Transplant.* 2002;17:1170–1175.

111. D'Haese PC, De Broe ME. Aluminum toxicity. In: Daugirdas JT, Ing TS, eds. *Handbook of Dialysis.* 2nd ed. Boston, Mass: Little Brown; 1994:522–536.

112. Kerr DNS, Ward MK, Ellis HA, Simpson W, Parkinson IS. Aluminum intoxication in renal disease. *Ciba Foundation Symposium.* 1992;169:123–141.

113. Alfrey AC. Aluminum toxicity in patients with chronic renal failure. *Ther Drug Monit.* 1993;15:593–597.

114. Ittel TH. Determinants of gastrointestinal absorption and distribution of aluminum in health and uremia. *Nephrol Dial Transplant.* 1993;8(Suppl 1):17–24.

115. The European Dialysis and Transplant Association—European Renal Association Consensus Conference. Diagnosis and treatment of aluminum overload in end-stage renal failure patients. *Nephrol Dial Transplant.* 1993;8(Suppl 1):1–4.

116. Jehle PM, Jehle DR, Mohan S, Keller F. Renal osteodystrophy: new insights in pathophysiology and treatment modalities with special emphasis on the insulin-like growth factor system. *Nephron.* 1998;79:249–264.

117. Lin JL, Lim PS, Leu ML. Relationship of body iron status and serum aluminum in chronic renal insufficiency patients not taking any aluminum-containing drugs. *Am J Nephrol.* 1995;15:118–122.

118. Cannata JB, Olaizola IR, Gomez-Alonso C, Menéndez-Fraga P, Alonso-Suarez M, Diaz-Lopez JB. Serum aluminum transport and aluminum uptake in chronic renal failure: role of iron and aluminum metabolism. *Nephron.* 1993;65:141–146.

119. Goodman WG. Diagnosis and treatment of aluminum-related bone disease. *Nephrology Exchange.* 1992;2:13–20.

120. Drüeke TB. Adynamic bone disease, anaemia, resistance to erythropoietin and iron-aluminum interaction. *Nephrol Dial Transplant.* 1993;8(Suppl 1):12–16.

121. Mucsi I, Hercz G. Adynamic bone disease: pathogenesis, diagnosis and clinical relevance. *Curr Opin Nephrol Hypertens.* 1997;7:356–361.

122. Kaye M. Bone disease. In: Daugirdas JT, Ing TS, eds. *Handbook of Dialysis.* 2nd ed. Boston, Mass: Little Brown; 1994:503–521.

123. Nestel AW, Meyers AM, Paiker J, Rollin HB. Effect of calcium supplement preparation containing small amounts of citrate on the absorption of aluminum in normal subjects and in renal failure patients. *Nephron.* 1994;68:197–201.

124. Lindberg JS, Copley JB, Koenig KG, Cushner HM. Effect of citrate on serum aluminum concentrations in hemodialysis patients: a prospective study. *South Med J.* 1993;86:1385–1388.

125. Nolan CR, Califano JR, Butzin CA. Influence of calcium acetate or calcium citrate on intestinal aluminum absorption. *Kidney Int.* 1990;38:937–941.

126. Yaqoob M, Ahmad R, McClelland P, Shivakumar KA, Sallomi DF, Fahal IH, Roberts NB, Helliwell T. Resistance to recombinant human erythropoietin due to aluminum overload and its reversal by low-dose desferrioxamine therapy. *Postgrad Med J*. 1993;69:124–128.

127. Davenport A, Davison AM, Will EJ, Newton KE, Toothill C. Aluminum mobilization following renal transplantation and the possible effect on susceptibility to bacterial sepsis. *Q J Med*. 1991;79:407–423.

128. Kausz AT, Antonsen JE, Hercz G, Pei Y, Weiss NS, Emerson S, Sherrard DJ. Screening plasma aluminum levels in relation to aluminum bone disease among asymptomatic dialysis patients. *Am J Kidney Dis*. 1999;34:688–693.

129. Levine DZ. *Care of the Renal Patient*. 2nd ed. Philadelphia, Pa: WB Saunders; 1991.

130. Boelaert JR, de Locht M. Side-Effects of desferrioxamine in dialysis patients. *Nephrol Dial Transplant*. 1993;8(Suppl 1):43–46.

131. NKF-K/DOQI clinical practice guidelines for anemia of chronic kidney disease: update 2000. *Am J Kidney Dis*. 2001;37(1 Suppl 1):S182–S238.

132. Hill LJ, Biesecker RL. Iron supplementation in dialysis patients with regard to cardiovascular disease and iron overload. *Top Clin Nutr*. 1996;12:41–50.

133. Fishbane S, Maesaka JK. Iron management in end-stage renal disease. *Am J Kidney Dis*. 1997;29:319–333.

134. Nissenson AR. Achieving target hematocrit in dialysis patients: new concepts in iron management. *Am J Kidney Dis*. 1997;30:907–911.

135. Hörl WH. Chairman's Workshop Report: is there a role for adjuvant therapy in patients being treated with epoetin? *Nephrol Dial Transplant*. 1999;14(Suppl 2):50–60.

136. Staab P. Back to basics: understanding iron balance in hemodialysis patients. *Renal Nutr Forum*. 1994;13:6–7.

137. Kooistra MP, Niemantsverdriet EC, van Es A, Mol-Beermann NM, Struyvenberg A, Marx JJM. Iron absorption in erythropoietin-treated haemodialysis patients: effects of iron availability, inflammation and aluminum. *Nephrol Dial Transplant*. 1998;13:82–88.

138. Sunder-Plassmann G, Hörl WH. Erythropoietin and iron. *Clin Nephrol*. 1997;47:141–157.

139. Drüeke TB, Bárány P, Cazzola M, Eschbach JW, Grützmacher P, Kaltwasser JP, MacDougall IC, Pippard MJ, Shaldon S, van Wyck D. Management of iron deficiency in renal anemia: guidelines for the optimal therapeutic approach in erythropoietin-treated patients. *Clin Nephrol*. 1997;48:1–8.

140. Eschbach JW. Current concepts of anemia management in chronic renal failure: impact of NKF-DOQI. *Semin Nephrol*. 2000;29:320–329.

141. Norton P. Advances in practice: trends in anemia management in patients with renal disease. *Renal Nutr Forum*. 2002;21:7–9.

142. MacDougall IC, Chandler G, Elston O, Harchowal J. Beneficial effects of adopting an aggressive intravenous iron policy in a hemodialysis unit. *Am J Kidney Dis*. 1999;34(4 Suppl 2):S40–S46.

143. Sunder-Plassmann G, Hörl WH. Safety aspects of parenteral iron in patients with end-stage renal disease. *Drug Saf*. 1997;17:241–250.

144. Kausz AT, Obrador GT, Pereira BJG. Anemia management in patients with chronic renal insufficiency. *Am J Kidney Dis*. 2000;36(6 Suppl 3):S39–S51.

145. Besarab A, Frinak S, Yee J. An indistinct balance: the safety and efficacy of parenteral iron therapy. *J Am Soc Nephrol*. 1999;10:2029–2043.

146. Bailie GR, Johnson CA, Mason NA. Parenteral iron use in the management of anemia in end-stage renal disease patients. *Am J Kidney Dis*. 2000;35:1–12.

147. Van Wyck DB, Cavallo G, Spinowitz BS, Adhikarla R, Gagnon S, Charytan C, Levin N. Safety and efficacy of iron sucrose in patients sensitive to iron dextran: North American clinical trial. *Am J Kidney Dis*. 2000;36:88–97.

148. Ifudu O. Parenteral Iron: Pharmacology and clinical use. *Nephron*. 1998;80:249–256.

149. Park L, Uhthoff T, Tierney M, Nadler S. Effect of an intravenous iron dextran regimen on iron stores, hemoglobin, and erythropoietin requirements in hemodialysis patients. *Am J Kidney Dis*. 1998;31:835–840.

150. Lindeman RD. Trace minerals and the kidney: an overview. *J Am Coll Nutr*. 1989;8:285–291.

151. Fishbane S. Iron treatment: impact of safety issues. *Am J Kidney Dis*. 1998;32(6 Suppl 4):S152–S156.

152. Van Wyck DB, Bailie G, Aronoff G. Just the FAQs: frequently asked questions about iron and anemia in patients with chronic kidney disease. *Am J Kidney Dis.* 2002;39:426–432.

153. Tarng DC, Wei YH, Huang TP, Kuo BIT, Yang WC. Intravenous ascorbic acid as an adjuvant therapy for recombinant erythropoietin in hemodialysis patients with hyperferritinemia. *Kidney Int.* 1999;55:2477–2486.

154. Mahajan SK. Zinc in kidney disease. *J Am Coll Nutr.* 1989;8:296–304.

155. Mahajan SK, Bowersox EM, Rye DL, Abu-Hamdan DK, Prasad AS, McDonald FD, Biersack KL. Factors underlying abnormal zinc metabolism in uremia. *Kidney Int.* 1989;36(Suppl 27):S269–S273.

156. Kelch E. Back to basics: do we need to think about zinc? *Renal Nutr Forum.* 1995;14:6–8.

157. Metcoff J. Guest editorial: nutrition in kidney disease. *J Am Coll Nutr.* 1989;8:267–270.

158. Melichar B, Aichberger C, Artner-Dworzak E, Weiss G, Margreiter R, Wachter H, Fuchs D. Immune activation and enhanced urinary zinc concentrations in allograft recipients. *Presse Med.* 1994;23:702–706.

159. Littlefield D. Zinc supplementation in wound healing of two hemodialysis patients, with alleviation of pruritus in the second. *Dial Transplant.* 1999;28:212–213.

160. Demling RH, DeBiasse MA. Micronutrients in critical illness. *Crit Care Clin.* 1995;11:651–673.

161. Braunschweig C. Minerals and trace elements. In: Matarese LE, Gottschlich MM. *Contemporary Nutrition Support Practice: A Clinical Guide.* Philadelphia, Pa: WB Saunders; 1998:163–173.

162. Baumgartner TG. Trace elements in clinical nutrition. *Nutr Clin Pract.* 1993;8:251–263.

163. Fosmire GJ. Zinc toxicity. *Am J Clin Nutr.* 1990;51:225–227.

164. Zima T, Mestek O, N?me?k K, Bártová V, Fialová J, Tesa? V, Suchánek M. Trace elements in hemodialysis and continuous ambulatory peritoneal dialysis patients. *Blood Purif.* 1998;16:253–260.

165. Lee SH, Huang JW, Hung KY, Leu LJ, Kan YT, Yang CS, Wu DC, Huang CL, Chen PY, Chen JS, Chen WY. Trace metals' abnormalities in hemodialysis patients: relationship with medications. *Artif Organs.* 2000;24:841–844.

166. Smith AM, Temple K. Selenium metabolism and renal disease. *J Ren Nutr.* 1997;7:69–72.

167. Girelli D, Olivieri O, Stanzial AM, Azzini M, Lupo A, Bernich P, Menini C, Gammaro L, Corrocher R. Low platelet glutathione peroxidase activity and serum selenium concentration in patients with chronic renal failure: relations to dialysis treatments, diet and cardiovascular complications. *Clin Sci.* 1993;84:611–617.

168. Saint-Georges MD, Bonnefont DJ, Bourely BA, Jaudon MCT, Cereze P, Chaumeil P, Gard C, D'Auzac CL. Correction of selenium deficiency in hemodialyzed patients. *Kidney Int.* 1989;36(Suppl 27):S274–S277.

169. Roxborough HE, Mercer C, McMaster D, Maxwell AP, Young IS. Plasma glutathione peroxidase activity is reduced in haemodialysis patients. *Nephron.* 1999;81:278–283.

170. Zachara BA, Adamowicz A, Trafikowska U, Pilecki D, Manitius J. Decreased plasma glutathione peroxidase activity in uremic patients. *Nephron.* 2000;84:278–279.

171. Food and Nutrition Board. *Recommended Dietary Allowances.* 10th ed. Washington, DC: National Academy Press; 1989.

172. Yilmaz ME, Kiraz M, Kara IH. The evaluation of serum zinc and copper levels in hemodialysis patients in southeast Turkey. *Dial Transplant.* 2000;29:718–720,746.

173. Brown ML, ed. *Present Knowledge in Nutrition.* 6th ed. Washington, DC: International Life Sciences Institute; 1990.

174. Romero RA, Salgado O, Rodriguez-Iturbe B, Tahan JE. Blood levels of chromium in diabetic and nondiabetic hemodialysis patients. *Transplant Proc.* 1996;28:3382–3384.

175. Gitelman HJ, Alderman FR, Perry SJ. Silicon accumulation in dialysis patients. *Am J Kidney Dis.* 1992;19:140–143.

Section 12
Physical Signs of Nutrient Deficiencies/Excesses

Body Area	Clinical Signs	Nutrient Considerations
Hair	• Dull, dry, brittle, sparse, shedding, or easily pluckable • Corkscrew, "swan-neck" deformity, perifollicular hemorrhages, follicular hyperkeratosis • Dyspigmentation	• Protein-energy malnutrition; zinc, biotin deficiencies • Vitamin C, vitamin A deficiencies • Biotin deficiency, protein-energy malnutrition
Skin	• Xerosis, follicular hyperkeratosis, mosaic dermatitis • Hyperpigmentation of skin • Petechiae, ecchymoses • Perifolliculosis • Pellagrous dermatitis • Seborrheic-like dermatitis • Flaky paint dermatosis, thin and inelastic • Poor wound healing, pressure sores • Thickening of pressure points (widespread)	• Vitamin A, essential fatty acid deficiencies • Protein-energy malnutrition; folate, vitamin B-12 deficiencies; carotene excess • Vitamin C, vitamin K deficiencies • Vitamin C deficiency • Niacin deficiency • Riboflavin, biotin, zinc, vitamin B-6, linoleic acid deficiencies • Protein-energy malnutrition • Protein, vitamin C, zinc, linoleic acid deficiencies • Niacin deficiency
Eyes	• Keratomalacia, Bitot's spots, conjunctival xerosis, corneal xerosis • Papilledema • Angular palpebritis • Corneal vascularization • Mild scleral icterus • Pallor of everted lower eyelids • Pale conjunctivae • Hollow look, dark circles, "sunken" eyes, loose skin, depleted fat pads	• Vitamin A deficiency • Vitamin A excess • Riboflavin, niacin deficiencies • Riboflavin deficiency • Pyridoxine deficiency • Iron, folate deficiencies • Iron, folate, vitamin B-12 deficiencies • Protein-energy malnutrition
Face and neck	• Nasolabial seborrhea • Distention or pulsation in neck veins • Goiter • Bilateral enlarged parotid glands	• Riboflavin, niacin, vitamin B-6 deficiencies • Fluid excess • Iodine deficiency • Protein deficiency

continues on next page

Body Area	Clinical Signs	Nutrient Considerations (continued)
Lips	• Cheilosis • Small ecchymotic lesions • Bilateral angular stomatitis • Pallor	• Riboflavin, vitamin B-6, niacin deficiencies • Protein-energy malnutrition; vitamin C, vitamin K deficiencies • Riboflavin, vitamin B-6, iron, niacin, zinc deficiencies • Iron deficiency
Gums	• Bleeding, red, swollen, or spongy • Red discoloration of gingiva • Inflammation with stomatitis and ulceration • Surface bald, smooth, beefy red • Pale gumline and oral mucosa	• Vitamin C deficiency • Vitamin A excess • Vitamin C, folate, vitamin B-12 deficiencies • Niacin deficiency • Iron deficiency
Tongue	• Smooth, pale, atrophic filiform papillae • Edema, fissuring • Lobulated with atrophy • Pallor and patchy atrophy • Magenta tongue, pebbly or granular dorsum • Scarlet, raw, and painful with atrophy • Glossitis • Taste atrophy	• Niacin, iron, vitamin B-12, folate, riboflavin deficiencies • Niacin deficiency • Folate deficiency • Biotin deficiency • Riboflavin, biotin deficiencies • Niacin, folate, vitamin B-12 deficiencies • Niacin, folate, riboflavin, iron, vitamin B-6, vitamin B-12, tryptophan deficiencies • Zinc, vitamin A deficiencies
Teeth	• Mottled enamel	• Fluorine excess
Nails	• Brittle, ridged, pale nail bed • Leukonychia • White spotting • Onycholysis • Paronychia, Beau's lines • Koilonychia • Bruising, bleeding • Splinter hemorrhages	• Iron deficiency • Zinc, niacin deficiencies • Zinc deficiency • Niacin, iron deficiencies • Zinc deficiency • Iron, zinc, copper, sulfur-containing amino acids deficiencies • Protein-energy malnutrition • Vitamin C deficiency
Hands	• Intraosseous atrophy	• Protein-energy malnutrition
Musculoskeletal	• Muscle wasting: deltoid and quadricep atrophy • Prominent bone structures: clavicles, ribs, shoulder, scapula, knee • Loss of subcutaneous fat over triceps, biceps, chest • Epiphyseal enlargement • Swollen, painful joints • Bowed legs • Beading of ribs • Pain in thighs, calves • Musculoskeletal hemorrhages	• Protein-energy malnutrition • Protein-energy malnutrition • Protein-energy malnutrition • Vitamin D, vitamin C deficiencies • Vitamin C deficiency • Vitamin D, calcium deficiencies • Vitamin D, calcium deficiencies • Thiamin deficiency • Vitamin C deficiency

continues on next page

Body Area	Clinical Signs	Nutrient Considerations (continued)
Neurologic	• Sensory loss, motor weakness, calf tenderness	• Thiamin deficiency
	• Ataxia	• Thiamin, vitamin E deficiencies; vitamin B-6 excess
	• Paresthesia	• Vitamin B-12 deficiency; vitamin B-6 excess
	• Weakness	• Protein-energy malnutrition; vitamin B-12 deficiency
	• Slow mentation, mental depression	• Protein-energy malnutrition; vitamin B-6, biotin deficiencies
	• Loss of vibratory sense, loss of ankle and knee-jerk reflexes	• Thiamin, vitamin B-12 deficiencies
	• Listlessness, apathy, mental confusion	• Protein deficiency
	• Tetany	• Calcium, magnesium deficiencies
	• Dementia	• Niacin, vitamin B-12 deficiencies

Bibliography

Enia G, Sicusco C, Alati G, Zoccali C. Subjective global assessment of nutrition in dialysis patients. *Nephrol Dial Transplant*. 1993;8:1094–1098.

Goldstein DJ. Assessment of nutrition status in renal diseases. In: Mitch WE, Klahr S, eds. *Handbook of Nutrition and the Kidney*. 3rd ed. Philadelphia, Pa: Lippincott-Raven Publishers; 1998:45–86.

Grant A, DeHoog S. *Nutritional Assessment and Support*. 5th ed. Seattle, Wash: Grant and DeHoog Publishers; 1999.

Jeejeebhoy KN, Detsky AS, Baker JP. Assessment of nutritional status. *JPEN J Parenter Enteral Nutr*. 1990;14(5 Suppl):193S-196S.

Kelly MP, Kight MA, Castillo S. Trophic implications of altered body composition observed in or near the nails of hemodialysis patients. *Adv Ren Replace Ther*. 1998;5:241–251.

Kelly MP, Kight MA, Rodriguez R, Castillo S. A diagnostically reasoned case study with particular emphasis on B6 and zinc imbalance directed by clinical history and nutrition physical examination findings. *Nutr Clin Pract*. 1998;13:32–39.

Matarese LE, Gottschlich MM. *Contemporary Nutrition Support Practice: A Clinical Guide*. Philadelphia, Pa: WB Saunders; 1998.

McCann L. Subjective global assessment as it pertains to the nutritional status of dialysis patients. *Dial Transplant*. 1996;25:190–199,202,225.

McCann L, ed. *Pocket Guide to Nutrition Assessment of the Renal Patient*. 3rd ed. New York, NY: National Kidney Foundation; 2002.

National Kidney Foundation Kidney Disease Outcome Quality Initiative Advisory Board. K/DOQI clinical practice guidelines for nutrition in chronic renal failure. Appendix VI. Methods for performing subjective global assessment. *Am J Kidney Dis*. 2000;35(6 Suppl 2):S75.

Zeman FJ. *Clinical Nutrition and Dietetics*. 2nd ed. New York, NY: Macmillan Publishing; 1991.

Section 13

Reasons for Inadequate Response to Erythropoietin

The most common cause of an incomplete response to erythropoietin (EPO) is iron deficiency (1). Prior to initiation of EPO therapy, the patient's iron status should be evaluated. In the iron-replete patient, the following conditions are possible causes for an inadequate response to EPO (1–9):

- Infection/inflammation
- Anemia of chronic disease
- Underdialysis
- Folate or vitamin B-12 deficiency
- Chronic blood loss (eg, gastrointestinal bleeding, frequent blood sampling, residual blood in dialyzer and blood lines, clotting of dialyzer)
- Secondary hyperparathyroidism/osteitis fibrosa
- Aluminum overload
- Sickle cell anemia
- Alpha and beta thalassemias
- Hemoglobinopathy
- Multiple myeloma
- Malignancy/immunosuppression
- Malnutrition
- Hemolysis
- Oxalosis (leading to bone marrow infiltration by oxalate crystals)
- Carnitine deficiency
- Angiotensin-converting enzyme (ACE) inhibitor use

References

1. NKF-K/DOQI clinical practice guidelines for anemia of chronic kidney disease: update 2000. *Am J Kidney Dis*. 2001;37(1 Suppl 1):S182–S238.

2. Fishbane S, Maesaka JK. Iron management in end-stage renal disease. *Am J Kidney Dis*. 1997;29:319–333.

3. Sunder-Plassmann G, Hörl WH. Erythropoietin and iron. *Clin Nephrol*. 1997;47:141–157.

4. Rao DS, Shih MS, Mohini R. Effect of serum parathyroid hormone and bone marrow fibrosis on the response to erythropoietin in uremia. *N Engl J Med*. 1993;328:171–175.

5. Hmida MB, Hachicha J, Kamoun K, Hamida N, Kaddour N, Bahloul A, Jlidi R, Jarraya A. Two cases of oxalosis as a cause of resistance to recombinant human erythropoietin. *Dial Transplant*. 1996;25:858–860,880.

6. Kopple JD, Massry SG, eds. *Nutritional Management of Renal Disease*. Baltimore, Md: Williams & Wilkins; 1997.

7. AAKP Carnitine Renal Dialysis Consensus Group. Role of L-carnitine in treating renal dialysis patients. *Dial Transplant*. 1994;23:177–181.

8. Kausz AT, Obrador GT, Pereira BJG. Anemia management in patients with chronic renal insufficiency. *Am J Kidney Dis*. 2000;36(6 Suppl 3):S39–S51.

9. Hörl WH. Is there a role for adjuvant therapy in patients being treated with epoetin? *Nephrol Dial Transplant*. 1999;14(Suppl 2):50–60.

Section 14
Glomerular Filtration Rate and Creatinine Clearance

The *Glomerular Filtration Rate* (GFR) is the best overall method for assessing renal function and determining level of therapy in patients with chronic kidney disease (CKD). Creatinine clearance (C_{cr}) has been the most commonly used method for measuring GFR, and several formulas have been developed to estimate creatinine clearance from serum creatinine levels. One of the formulas that have been used widely is the Cockcroft-Gault equation (1):

Formula 1: $C_{cr} \text{ (mL/min)} = \dfrac{(140 - \text{Age}) \times \text{Wt}}{72 \times \text{Ser Cr}} \times (0.85 \text{ if female})$

Where:

> Ser Cr = serum creatinine (mg/dL)
> Wt = weight (kg)
> Age is measured in years

The calculated clearance from this equation should be multiplied by 0.80 for patients with paraplegia and by 0.60 for quadriplegia (2,3).

Example: For a 50-year-old woman weighing 68 kg with a creatinine of 2.1 mg/dL:

$$C_{cr} \text{ (mL/min)} = \frac{(140 - 50) \times 68}{72 \times 2.1} \times (0.85) = 34.4 \text{ mL/min}$$

If the woman were a paraplegic, then the estimated creatinine clearance would be:

$$C_{cr} \text{ (mL/min)} = \frac{(140 - 50) \times 68}{72 \times 2.1} \times (0.85) \times (0.80) = 27.5 \text{ mL/min}$$

A formula based on data from 1,070 subjects enrolled in the Modification of Diet in Renal Disease (MDRD) study has been published and shown to be a more accurate estimate of GFR than other commonly used equations, including the Cockcroft-Gault equation (4). The equation predicts GFR directly, rather than from creatinine clearance, and provides the result standardized for body surface area (4). It is accurate up to a value of approximately 90 mL/min/1.73 m^2 (4,5).

Formula 2: $\text{GFR (mL/min/1.73 m}^2) = 170 \times (\text{Ser CR})^{-0.999} \times (\text{Age})^{-0.176} \times (0.762) \text{ (if female)}$
$\times (1.180) \text{ (if African American)} \times (\text{BUN})^{-0.170} \times (\text{Alb})^{0.318}$

Where:

> Ser Cr = serum creatinine (mg/dL)
> BUN = blood urea nitrogen (mg/dL)

Alb = serum albumin (g/dL)
Age is measured in years

Example: Consider the same 50-year-old woman from the previous example, not African American, with an albumin of 3.8, a serum creatinine of 2.1, and BUN of 25:

$$\text{GFR (mL/min/1.73 m}^2) = 170 \times (2.1)^{-0.999} \times (50)^{-0.176} \times (0.762) \times (25)^{-0.170} \times (3.8)^{0.318}$$
$$= 170 \times (0.477) \times (0.502) \times (0.762) \times (0.579) \times (1.529) = 27.5 \text{ mL/min/1.73 m}^2$$

An abbreviated form of the MDRD equation using only 4 variables has been developed and shown to be similar in accuracy to the original equation (5). This equation is recommended by the National Kidney Foundation K/DOQI Clinical Practice Guidelines for Chronic Kidney Disease (5).

Formula 3: $\text{GFR (mL/min/1.73 m}^2) = 186 \times (\text{Ser Cr})^{-1.154} \times (\text{Age})^{-0.203} \times (0.742)$ (if female)
$\times (1.21)$ (if African American)

Where:

Ser Cr = serum creatinine (mg/dL)
Age is measured in years

Example: Consider the same woman above, using Formula 3 to determine GFR:

$$\text{GFR (mL/min/1.73 m}^2) = 186 \times (2.1)^{-1.154} \times (50)^{-0.203} \times 0.742$$
$$= 186 \times (0.425) \times (0.452) \times (0.742) = 26.5 \text{ mL/min/1.73 m}^2$$

The formulas presented are not accurate for patients who are not in a steady state of creatinine balance, such as patients with acute renal failure, patients in a catabolic state and whose muscle mass is being destroyed, and patients receiving dialysis (2,4,5). Other situations in which estimates of creatinine clearance or GFR may be inaccurate include unusually high or low muscle mass, unusually high or low creatine intake (eg, use of creatine supplements or vegetarian diet, respectively), extremes of age and body size, severe malnutrition or obesity, diseases of skeletal muscle, or use of drugs that interfere with creatinine secretion (eg, cimetidine or trimethoprim) (4,5). For these patients, actual clearance should be measured using a timed urine collection (4,5).

References

1. Cockcroft DW, Gault MH. Prediction of creatinine clearance from serum creatinine. *Nephron.* 1976;16:31–41.

2. Daugirdas JT, Ing TS, eds. *Handbook of Dialysis.* 3rd ed. Boston, Mass: Little Brown; 2000.

3. McCann L, ed. *Pocket Guide to Nutrition Assessment of the Renal Patient.* 3rd ed. New York, NY: National Kidney Foundation; 2002.

4. Levey AS, Bosch JP, Lewis JB, Greene T, Rogers N, Roth D. A more accurate method to estimate glomerular filtration rate from serum creatinine: a new prediction equation. Modification of Diet in Renal Disease Study Group. *Ann Intern Med.* 1999;130:461–470.

5. National Kidney Foundation Kidney Disease Outcome Quality Initiative Advisory Board. K/DOQI clinical practice guidelines for chronic kidney disease: evaluation, classification, and stratification. Guideline 4. Estimation of GFR. *Am J Kidney Dis.* 2002;39(2 Suppl 1):S76–S119.

Section 15

Protein Catabolic Rate and Protein Equivalent of Nitrogen Appearance Rate

Protein Catabolic Rate (PCR) is a term that traditionally has been used to represent the net rate of protein breakdown based on the urea generation rate. Because urea is the major component of nitrogen excretion, which varies with protein intake, PCR has been used to provide an estimate of protein intake or needs. PCR, however, actually represents the net amount of protein catabolism beyond the amount of protein synthesis in the body (1). The true protein catabolic rate is about 6 times more than PCR estimated from urea generation rate, because most of the catabolized protein is not catabolized to urea but used again for protein synthesis (2). For this reason, the term *Protein Equivalent of Nitrogen Appearance Rate* (PNA) has been suggested as a more accurate term.

The formulas for PCR do not factor in other protein losses that may occur, such as urinary or dialysate protein losses, which can be substantial in some renal patients, especially those on peritoneal dialysis. The PNA, however, has been defined to include these extra losses and is thus a more accurate reflection of what is being measured (3). In patients with no direct protein losses, the PNA is equal to PCR (1). In patients with substantial urinary or dialytic protein losses, the direct protein losses must be added to the PCR to yield the true PNA (1,3). In many cases, the term *PNA* is used for calculation with peritoneal dialysis patients and *PCR* is used with non-dialysis and hemodialysis patients (assumed to have no extraneous protein losses).

Formulas for calculating PNA and PCR are presented in this section. Additional formulas for determining PCR in hemodialysis patients using Kt/V appear in the Dialysis Adequacy section (Section 16).

PNA can be estimated directly from urea nitrogen appearance (UNA). UNA is the amount of urea nitrogen that appears in body fluids and all outputs (eg, urine, dialysate, fistula drainage) plus the change in the body stores of urea nitrogen. Formulas to calculate UNA appear at the end of this section.

For **non-dialyzed or hemodialysis patients** without substantial urinary protein losses, PNA is equal to PCR and can be calculated using Formula 1 (1).

Formula 1: PCR(g/day) = (6.49 × UNA) + (0.294 × V)

Where:

> V = total body water volume (L) and can be calculated using the volume equations in Section 17.

If **substantial urinary or dialytic protein losses are present** (> 0.1 g/kg), direct protein losses must be added to the PCR to yield the true PNA (1).

Formula 2: PNA = PCR + protein losses

For **peritoneal dialysis patients,** PNA can be estimated by (1):

Formula 3: PNA(g/day) = $10.76 \times [(0.69 \times UNA) + 1.46]$

- This equation assumes a mean dialysate protein loss of 7.3 g/day and is useful if dialysate protein losses cannot be measured.
- High-transport patients (those patients who have high transport rates of small solutes across the peritoneal membrane) may lose more protein into dialysate than other peritoneal dialysis patients (1). In these patients, it is best to measure protein losses in dialysate directly, and if dialysate protein losses exceed 15 g/day, calculate PNA as PCR plus urinary and dialytic protein losses (1) (Formula 2).

Bergström has also developed formulas for estimating PNA in **peritoneal dialysis patients** using UNA (4).

Formula 4: PNA (g/day) = $15.1 + (6.95 \times UNA) +$ protein losses

When urinary and protein losses cannot be measured, the following formula can be used. It should not be used, however, if protein losses are high (1,4).

Formula 5: PNA (g/day) = $20.1 + (7.50 \times UNA)$

PNA is often adjusted or "normalized" to lean (ie, fat-free and edema-free) body mass and is expressed as *nPNA* (5).

Formula 6: nPNA (g/day/kg body wt) = $\dfrac{PNA}{[V/0.58]}$

Where:
    V = total body water volume (L) (see Section 17)
    0.58 = percent of lean body mass assumed to contain water

The following are additional formulas that may be used in **peritoneal dialysis patients** to determine PNA from urea appearance (UA). The Randerson equation has been the most widely used (6). The Bergström equations, however, are more recently published and are based on nitrogen balance studies (6). They may thus be better for assessing adequacy of protein intake (6).

Randerson Equation (6)

Formula 7: PNA (g/24hr) = $(0.19 \times UA) + 8$

Bergström Equations (2,6,7)

For use when urea appearance and protein losses have been calculated:

Formula 8: PNA (g/24hr) = $(0.261 \times UA) + 13 +$ protein losses

For use in the absence of excessive protein losses:

Formula 9: $PNA(g/24hr) = (0.272 \times UA) + 19$

Where:

UA = urea appearance in the dialysate and urine (mmol/24hrs)

protein losses = protein losses in urine and drained dialysate (g/24 hr)

Urea Nitrogen Appearance

Nitrogen losses and nitrogen balance can be estimated from the *Urea Nitrogen Appearance* (UNA). UNA is the amount of urea nitrogen that appears in body fluids and all outputs (eg, urine, dialysate, fistula drainage) plus the change in the body stores of urea nitrogen.

Formula 10: $UNA(g/day) = UUN + DUN + \text{Change in BUN}$

Where:

UUN = Urinary urea nitrogen (measured from a 24 hr urine collection) (g/day)

DUN = Dialysate urea nitrogen (measured from the collection of dialysate outflow over 24 hr) (g/day)

Formula 11: $\text{Change in BUN}(g/day) = [(BUN_2 - BUN_1) \times 0.6 \times BW_1] + [(BW_2 - BW_1) \times BUN_2]$

Where:

BUN_1 = initial blood urea nitrogen (g/L)

BUN_2 = final blood urea nitrogen (g/L)

BW_1 = initial body weight (kg)

BW_2 = final body weight (kg)

0.6 = estimate of the fraction of body weight that is body water. This estimate may have to be increased in patients who are edematous or lean, and decreased in the obese.

For hemodialysis patients, BUN_1 is typically the post-dialysis BUN from the first hemodialysis session and BUN_2 is the pre-dialysis BUN from the subsequent session.

For patients who are not on dialysis, DUN equals zero. In hemodialysis patients and other intermittent dialysis patients, concentration of urea nitrogen in dialysate is low and difficult to measure, so the UNA is usually calculated during the interdialytic period. DUN then also becomes zero.

The time interval for the collection of the parameters of UNA is typically 24 hours. However, any time interval (eg, the entire interdialytic period) can be used as long as the same time interval is used for all the parameters (UUN, DUN, and initial and final BUNs and BWs). If desired, UNA can then be adjusted to a 24-hour period and reported as g/day instead of, for example, g/48 hours.

References

1. NKF-K/DOQI clinical practice guidelines for peritoneal dialysis adequacy: update 2000. *Am J Kidney Dis.* 2001;37(1 Suppl 1):S65–S136.
2. Heimbürger O, Bergström J, Lindholm B. Maintenance of optimal nutrition in CAPD. *Kidney Int.* 1994;46(Suppl 48):S39–S46.
3. Bargman JM. The rationale and ultimate limitations of urea kinetic modeling in the estimation of nutritional status. *Peritoneal Dial Int.* 1996;16:347–351.
4. Bergström J, Heimberger O, Lindholm B. Calculation of protein equivalent of total nitrogen appearance from urea appearance: which formulas should be used? *Perit Dial Int.* 1998;18:467–473.

5. National Kidney Foundation Kidney Disease Outcome Quality Initiative Advisory Board. K/DOQI clinical practice guidelines for nutrition in chronic renal failure. Guideline 8. Protein equivalent of total nitrogen appearance (PNA). *Am J Kidney Dis.* 2000;35(6 Suppl 2):S28–S29.

6. Krediet RT, Koomen GCM, Struijk DG, van Olden RW, Imholz ALT, Boeschoten EW. Practical methods for assessing dialysis efficiency during peritoneal dialysis. *Kidney Int.* 1994;46(Suppl 48):S7–S13.

7. Kopple JD, Massry SG, eds. *Nutritional Management of Renal Disease.* Baltimore, Md: Williams & Wilkins; 1997.

Section 16
Dialysis Adequacy

Adequacy of dialysis is defined through the use of urea kinetic modeling. The most abundant solute removed by dialysis is urea, an end-product of protein metabolism. Although urea is only mildly toxic and cannot account for most of the signs and symptoms observed in patients with renal failure, it does serve as a marker for other easily removed toxins. Kinetic modeling is the mathematical representation of the change of a substance over time, and urea kinetic modeling is the mathematical description of the generation and removal of urea in the chronic kidney disease (CKD) patient. By modeling this change in urea, practitioners can measure the dose of dialysis a patient is receiving and determine how well a patient is being dialyzed. Protein intake is also often estimated using urea kinetic modeling via the protein catabolic rate (PCR). Specifics behind the calculations for PCR are presented in Section 15, and formulas estimating PCR from kinetic modeling parameters appear later in this section.

Urea and the other toxins that accumulate in the blood in patients with kidney failure can diminish patient appetite, intake, and nutritional status. In the CKD (predialysis) patient, toxins accumulate, often causing altered taste and anorexia. Inadequate dialysis also often leads to anorexia and decreased intake and may be an important influence on nutritional status in the dialysis patient (1). In patients undergoing dialysis treatment, insufficient solute clearance may lead to accumulation of toxins, leading to nausea, anorexia, and weight loss, and insufficient ultrafiltration may also contribute to anorexia due to bowel-wall edema (2). Dietitians should monitor a patient's dialysis adequacy to determine if inadequate dialysis leading to toxin accumulation may be contributing to decreased nutrient intake.

Some studies have demonstrated a relationship between dialysis adequacy and nutritional status, but the extent of this relationship is controversial. The studies that have shown a positive correlation between dose of dialysis (as measured by Kt/V) and PCR have primarily been retrospective or cross-sectional and thus cannot demonstrate a cause-and-effect relationship between dialysis adequacy and protein or nutritional status (3,4). In fact, some speculate that the relationship found in these studies between Kt/V and PCR is actually a consequence of mathematical coupling rather than a true metabolic response, and the increase in PCR with increasing Kt/V may not represent a true increase in nutritional intake (3–6). The Canada-USA (CANUSA) Peritoneal Dialysis Study showed a positive correlation between change in dialysis dose and change in nutritional status, lending support to the contention that improved dialysis adequacy contributes to improved nutritional status (7). Additionally, results from a recent small prospective study suggested that increasing dialysis adequacy led to a positive effect on PCR and nutritional status (8). Although toxin accumulation can affect nutritional intake and status, it still is not clear whether and to what extent increasing dose of dialysis will improve nutritional status.

Determining Adequacy in Hemodialysis

In hemodialysis, two parameters are used to determine adequacy of dialysis: urea reduction ratio (URR) and Kt/V.

URR is defined as the percent reduction in urea concentration during the dialysis treatment. It is calculated as:

Formula 1: $URR\ (\%) = \left[1 - \left[\dfrac{Post - BUN}{Pre - BUN} \right] \right] \times 100$

Where:

Pre-BUN = blood urea nitrogen level before hemodialysis treatment (mg/dL)

Post-BUN = blood urea nitrogen level after hemodialysis treatment (mg/dL)

Kt/V is another method for modeling urea kinetics. In this model, "K" represents the dialyzer urea clearance in liters per minute, "t" is the dialysis time in minutes, and "V" is the volume of urea distribution in the body in liters (measured as the total body water volume). It is essentially a unitless term that factors the intensity of dialysis (K × t) by the patient's size (V) (9). Kt/V is most accurately determined through formal urea kinetic modeling calculated by computer programs. Many software packages will calculate Kt/V using this complicated set of formulas. More simplified equations can estimate Kt/V with a calculator. The most widely recommended formula is the natural logarithmic formula developed by Daugirdas (10).

Formula 2: $Kt/V = -Ln[R - (0.008 \times t)] + [4 - (3.5 \times R)] \times \left(\dfrac{UF}{Wt} \right)$

Where:

Ln = the natural logarithm

R = Post-BUN divided by Pre-BUN

t = dialysis session length (hr)

UF = ultrafiltration volume (L)

Wt = patient's post-dialysis weight (kg)

This formula assumes that the pool of urea is contained in a perfectly equilibrated single pool (11,12). This assumption is inaccurate, however, because a disequilibrium in urea concentration occurs during hemodialysis. Tissues that receive lower blood flows are unable to lose urea to the vascular space at a sufficient rate to maintain urea equilibrium. By the end of dialysis, these tissues will contain a higher concentration of urea than the blood. The urea in the tissues will eventually flow into the vascular space, leading to an increase in blood urea levels. This "urea rebound" may occur up to an hour after dialysis. As a result of this urea rebound, the efficiency of dialysis is less than that predicted by the previous single-pool formula, leading to an overestimation of dialysis adequacy (12). An adjustment to the formula corrects for the disequilibrium in the urea pool, and has been validated during the pilot trial for the Hemodialysis (HEMO) study (11,12).

Formula 3: $Kt/V_{equil} = Kt/V * \left[1 - \left[\dfrac{0.6}{t} \right] \right] + 0.03$

Where:

Kt/V = single pool Kt/V (Formula 2)

t = dialysis session length (hr)

Sources of Error

Certain factors can lead to errors in the estimation of the dose of dialysis. These include the following, which are discussed in more detail in the National Kidney Foundation Kidney Disease Outcome Quality Initiative (NKF-K/DOQI) Clinical Practice Guidelines for Hemodialysis Adequacy (13):

Factors That May Affect Urea Clearance (K)

- Access recirculation
- Inadequate blood flow from the vascular access

- Inaccurate estimation of dialyzer performance
- Inadequate dialyzer reprocessing
- Dialyzer clotting
- Air in dialyzer
- Blood pump/dialysate flow calibration inaccuracies
- Low dialysate flow rate
- Dialyzer leaks

Factors That May Affect Time (t)

- Decrease in dialysis treatment time (eg, due to clock errors, staff errors, patient request)
- Interruptions during dialysis session (eg, alarms, patient disconnections)
- Time on dialysis calculated inaccurately
- Error in documentation of time

Factors That May Affect Volume (V)

- Inaccuracies in weight and/or anthropometric data
- Blood sampling errors (timing and/or technique in pre- and post-dialysis BUNs—see Section 8)
- Laboratory error in processing or reporting
- Obesity
- Amputation (see Section 17 for adjusting volume for amputation)

An extensive algorithm is provided in the NKF-K/DOQI Hemodialysis Adequacy Guidelines for determining possible sources of error when a deficiency in the delivered Kt/V or URR occurs (13).

Twice-Weekly Hemodialysis

The information presented regarding dialysis dose and Kt/V is for hemodialysis performed 3 times weekly. When using formulas and computer programs to determine Kt/V in a twice-weekly situation, the Kt/V result obtained can be adjusted to reflect what the Kt/V would be if the patient were receiving that dose of dialysis 3 times per week (Kt/V_3).

Formula 4: $Kt/V_3 = \dfrac{Kt/V}{3} \times 2$

Calculation of nPCR

Determination of nPCR in hemodialysis patients requires measurement of urea generation, typically between two dialysis sessions. To calculate urea generation, a post-dialysis BUN from one dialysis session and a pre-dialysis BUN from a subsequent dialysis session are usually drawn. Kinetic modeling calculations, however, use a pre-dialysis BUN and post-dialysis BUN from the same dialysis session. To avoid the need to draw a third BUN, "two-BUN" formulas have been developed to estimate nPCR from the pre-dialysis BUN and the calculated Kt/V (14). These formulas are applicable to patients without significant residual renal function. All of the two-BUN equations have the following form (14):

Formula 5: $nPCR = \dfrac{Pre - BUN}{\left[a + b(Kt/V) + \left[\dfrac{c}{Kt/V} \right] \right]} + 0.168$

Where:

Pre-BUN = blood urea nitrogen level before hemodialysis treatment (mg/dL)

Kt/V = Kt/V calculated from the pre-dialysis and post-dialysis BUNs (see Formula 2)

The coefficients a, b, and c vary according to the day of the week that the pre-dialysis BUN is drawn and how frequently a patient receives dialysis. Tables 16.1 and 16.2 contain the numbers that are inserted for a, b, and c in Formula 4 depending on the day of the week that the pre-dialysis BUN is drawn (14). Table 16.1 is for dialysis 3 times per week, and Table 16.2 is for dialysis twice a week.

Table 16.1   Coefficients for Thrice-Weekly Dialysis

	a	b	c
Beginning of the week	36.3	5.48	53.5
Midweek	25.8	1.15	56.4
End of the week	16.3	4.30	56.6

Table 16.2   Coefficients for Twice-Weekly Dialysis

	a	b	c
Beginning of the week	48.0	5.14	79.0
End of the week	33.0	3.60	83.2

Residual Renal Function

Some patients continue to have a certain amount of residual renal function that helps to clear urea from the blood in addition to the clearance provided by dialysis. This residual function can be taken into account when determining dialysis adequacy, although it is not always recommended to do so in hemodialysis patients because residual renal function can deteriorate quickly (15). Residual renal clearance of urea (Kru) can be determined using the techniques listed in the following section , and the dialysis Kt/V can be adjusted to account for clearance provided by the kidneys, yielding a corrected Kt/V (Kt/V_{corr}) (see Formula 8).

Determination of Residual Renal Clearance of Urea (Kru) (15)

The patient is instructed to collect all urine between the end of one dialysis session and the start of the subsequent dialysis session. The patient is to start the urine collection by emptying his or her bladder after the first dialysis session, not saving the urine. All urine is then to be collected up to the next dialysis session and must be kept refrigerated. The patient is also instructed to empty his or her bladder right before the second dialysis session and to add this urine to the collected urine. At the end of the first dialysis, a post-dialysis BUN is drawn. A pre-dialysis BUN is drawn at the beginning of the next dialysis session. The mean urea nitrogen level in the blood between the dialysis sessions (BUN_{avg}) is then calculated (Formula 6) and used to calculate Kru (Formula 7).

Formula 6: Mean blood urea nitrogen (BUN) level

$$BUN_{avg}(mg/dL) = \frac{\text{post-dialysis BUN + pre-dialysis BUN}}{2}$$

Where:

post-dialysis BUN = BUN drawn at the end of the first dialysis session (mg/dL)
pre-dialysis BUN = BUN drawn at the start of the next dialysis session (mg/dL)

Formula 7: $\text{Kru(mL/min)} = \dfrac{V_u}{T} \times \dfrac{\text{UUN}}{\text{BUN}_{avg}}$

Where:

V_u = Volume of urine (mL)

T = Time of urine collection (ie, time between dialysis sessions) (min)

UUN = Urine urea nitrogen (mg/dL)

Calculation of Kt/V corrected for Kru (15):

Formula 8: For dialysis 3 times weekly:

$$\text{Kt/V}_{corr} = \text{Kt/V} + (5.5 \times \text{Kru/V})$$

For dialysis 2 times weekly:

$$\text{Kt/V}_{corr} = \text{Kt/V} + (9.5 \times \text{Kru/V})$$

Where:

V = Total body water volume (L)*

Kt/V = Dialysis Kt/V result

Determination of nPCR (14)

In calculating residual renal function, a post-dialysis BUN is used from the first hemodialysis session and a pre-dialysis BUN from a subsequent session is drawn. Because this second-session pre-dialysis BUN is known, the nPCR can be calculated using the urea nitrogen appearance (UNA)-based formulas in Section 15. The nPCR can also be determined for patients with significant residual function using the two-BUN formula for nPCR (Formula 5) (14). The pre-dialysis BUN from the first dialysis session (pre-BUN in Formula 5) must be adjusted upward (to pre-BUN$_{adj}$) before it is used in the two-BUN formula (see Formula 10) (14).

Formula 9: For dialysis 3 times weekly:

$$\text{Pre-BUN}_{adj} = \text{Pre-BUN} \times \left[1 + \left[0.70 + \left[\frac{3.08}{\text{Kt/V}} \right] \right] \times \frac{\text{Kru}}{\text{V}} \right]$$

For dialysis 2 times weekly:

$$\text{Pre-BUN}_{adj} = \text{Pre-BUN} \times \left[1 + \left[1.15 + \left[\frac{4.56}{\text{Kt/V}} \right] \right] \times \frac{\text{Kru}}{\text{V}} \right]$$

Where:

Pre-BUN_{adj} = Adjusted pre-dialysis BUN (mg/dL)

Pre-BUN = blood urea nitrogen level before the first dialysis treatment (mg/dL)

Kt/V = Dialysis Kt/V result

Kru = Residual renal clearance of urea (mL/min)

V = Total body water volume (L) (see Section 17)

The nPCR adjusted for residual function is then:

Formula 10: $\text{Adjusted nPCR} = \dfrac{\text{Pre-BUN}_{adj}}{\left[a + b(\text{Kt/V}) + \left[\dfrac{c}{\text{Kt/V}} \right] \right]} + 0.168$

Determining Adequacy in Peritoneal Dialysis

Total weekly creatinine clearance and total weekly Kt/V are measured to determine adequacy in peritoneal dialysis. The NKF-K/DOQI Clinical Practice Guidelines for Peritoneal Dialysis Adequacy recommend that measurements be taken when the patient is clinically stable (eg, stable weight, stable BUN and creatinine concentrations) and at least 4 weeks after resolution of peritonitis (16).

Total Weekly Creatinine Clearance

Total weekly creatinine clearance (Total C_{cr}) is determined as the sum of the residual renal C_{cr} and the dialysis C_{cr}. The NKF-K/DOQI Guidelines recommend calculating the glomerular filtration rate (GFR) as the mean of urea clearance (C_u) and creatinine clearance (C_{cr}) and using the GFR in place of the residual renal C_{cr} to correct for secretion of creatinine by the kidneys (16). Measurements of residual renal function should be taken every 6 to 12 months because residual renal function diminishes progressively with time, requiring an increase in dialysis to compensate (17).

Formula 11: $\text{Renal } C_{cr} \text{ (mL/min)} = \dfrac{\text{Urine creatinine}}{\text{Serum creatinine}} \times \dfrac{\text{Urine volume}}{\text{Collection time}}$

Where:

        Urine and serum creatinine are measured in mg/dL
        Urine volume is measured in mL
        Collection time is measured in min

Formula 12: $\text{Renal } C_u \text{ (mL/min)} = \dfrac{\text{UUN}}{\text{BUN}} \times \dfrac{\text{Urine volume}}{\text{Collection time}}$

Where:

        UUN = Urine urea nitrogen (mg/dL)
        BUN = Blood urea nitrogen (mg/dL)
        Volume and collection time are measured as above

Formula 13: $\text{GFR (mL/min)} = (\text{Renal } C_{cr} + \text{Renal } C_u)/2$

Formula 14: $\text{Dialysis } C_{cr} \text{ (mL/min)} = \dfrac{\text{Dialysate creatinine}}{\text{Serum creatinine}} \times \dfrac{\text{Dialysate drain volume}}{\text{Collection time}}$

Where:

        Dialysate and serum creatinine are measured in mg/dL
        Dialysate drain volume is measured in mL
        Collection time = Length of time of dialysate drainage collection (min)

Formula 15: $\text{Total } C_{cr} \text{ (mL/min)} = \text{GFR} + \text{Dialysis } C_{cr}$

Formula 16: $\text{Weekly Total } C_{cr} \text{ (L/wk)} = \dfrac{(\text{Total } C_{cr}) \times 10{,}080 \text{ min/wk}}{1{,}000 \text{ mL/L}}$

The NKF-K/DOQI Peritoneal Dialysis Adequacy Guidelines recommend normalizing the Weekly Total C_{cr} to 1.73 m^2 of body surface area (BSA) (16). Formulas for calculating BSA are available in Section 17.

Formula 17: $\text{Normalized Weekly Total } C_{cr} \text{ (L/wk/1.73 } m^2) = \dfrac{(\text{Weekly Total } C_{cr}) \times 1.73 m^2}{\text{Patient's BSA}}$

Total Weekly Kt/V

Total urea clearance (Total C_u) is first calculated from the sum of the residual renal urea clearance (Renal C_u) (see Formula 12 in this section) and the dialysis urea clearance (Dialysis C_u). This sum is then converted to weekly total urea clearance (Weekly Total C_u), as was done in the earlier example for creatinine clearance, and divided by total body water volume.

Formula 18: $\text{Dialysis } C_u = \dfrac{\text{Dialysate urea}}{\text{BUN}} \times \dfrac{\text{Dialysate drain volume}}{\text{Collection time}}$

Where:

Dialysate urea and BUN (blood urea nitrogen) are measured in mg/dL
Dialysate drain volume is measured in mL
Collection time = Length of time of dialysate drainage collection (min)

Formula 19: $\text{Total } C_u (\text{mL/min}) = \text{Renal } C_u + \text{Dialysis } C_u$

Formula 20: $\text{Weekly Total } C_u (\text{L/wk}) = \dfrac{(\text{Total } C_u) \times 10{,}080 \text{ min/wk}}{1{,}000 \text{ mL/L}}$

Formula 21: $\text{Weekly Kt/V} = \dfrac{\text{Weekly Total } C_u}{V}$

Where:

V = Total body water volume (L) (see Section 17)

Adequacy Recommendations

The NKF-K/DOQI Hemodialysis and Peritoneal Dialysis Adequacy Guidelines have suggested that the data in Table 16.3 be used as targets for determining adequacy (13,16,18):

Table 16.3   Adequacy Recommendations

Type of Dialysis	Kt/V	URR	Creatinine Clearance
Hemodialysis	Prescribed ≥ 1.3 Delivered ≥ 1.2	Prescribed ≥ 70% Delivered ≥ 65%	N/A*
Peritoneal Dialysis: CAPD	2.0 (weekly)	N/A	50 L/wk/1.73 m²—low and low-average transporters 60 L/wk/1.73 m²—high and high-average transporters
NIPD	2.2 (weekly)	N/A	66 L/wk/1.73 m²
CCPD	2.1 (weekly)	N/A	63 L/wk/1.73 m²
*N/A = Not applicable			

It has also been suggested that the Kt/V target for twice-weekly hemodialysis be approximately 1.8–2.0, which corresponds to a 3-times-weekly Kt/V of 1.2–1.3 (15).

Adjustment for Amputation

If a patient has an amputation, volume and body surface area (BSA) need to be adjusted before use in the equations for determining dialysis adequacy. More information about adjusting volume and BSA for amputations is available in Section 17.

References

1. Wolfson M. Causes, manifestations, and assessment of malnutrition in chronic renal failure. In: Kopple JD, Massry SG, eds. *Nutritional Management of Renal Disease.* Baltimore, Md: Williams & Wilkins; 1997:245–256.

2. Chertow GM, Bullard A, Lazarus JM. Nutrition and the dialysis prescription. *Am J Nephrol.* 1996;16:79–89.

3. Ikizler TA, Schulman G. Adequacy of dialysis. *Kidney Int.* 1997;52(Suppl 62):S96–S100.

4. Ahmed KR, Kopple JD. Nutrition in maintenance hemodialysis patients. In: Kopple JD, Massry SG, eds. *Nutritional Management of Renal Disease.* Baltimore, Md: Williams & Wilkins, 1997:563–600.

5. Stein A, Walls J. The correlation between Kt/V and protein catabolic rate—a self-fulfilling prophecy. *Nephrol Dial Transplant.* 1994;9:743–745.

6. Harty J, Venning M, Gokal R. Does CAPD guarantee adequate dialysis delivery and nutrition? *Nephrol Dial Transplant.* 1994;9:1721–1723.

7. McCusker FX, Teehan BP, Thorpe KE, Keshaviah PR, Churchill DN. How much peritoneal dialysis is required for the maintenance of a good nutritional status? *Kidney Int.* 1996;50(Suppl 56):S56–S61.

8. Marcus RG, Cohl E, Uribarri J. Protein intake seems to respond to increases in Kt/V despite baseline Kt/V greater than 1.2. *Am J Nephrol.* 1999;19:500–504.

9. Depner TA. Urea modeling: the basics. *Semin Dial.* 1991;4:179–184.

10. Daugirdas JT. Second-generation logarithmic estimates of single-pool variable volume Kt/V: an analysis of error. *J Am Soc Nephrol.* 1993;4:1205–1213.

11. Daugirdas JT. Simplified equations for monitoring Kt/V, PCRn, eKt/V, and ePCRn. *Adv Ren Replace Ther.* 1995;2:295–304.

12. Depner T, Beck G, Daugirdas J, Kusek J, Eknoyan G. Lessons from the hemodialysis (HEMO) study: an improved measure of the actual hemodialysis dose. *Am J Kidney Dis.* 1999;3:142–149.

13. NKF-K/DOQI clinical practice guidelines for hemodialysis adequacy: update 2000. *Am J Kidney Dis.* 2001;37(1 Suppl 1):S7–S64.

14. Depner TA, Daugirdas JT. Equations for normalized protein catabolic rate based on two-point modeling of hemodialysis urea kinetics. *J Am Soc Nephrol.* 1996;7:780–785.

15. Daugirdas JT. Chronic hemodialysis prescription: a urea kinetic approach. In: Daugirdas JT, Ing TS, eds. *Handbook of Dialysis.* 2nd ed. Boston, Mass: Little Brown; 1994:92–120.

16. NKF-K/DOQI clinical practice guidelines for peritoneal dialysis adequacy: update 2000. *Am J Kidney Dis.* 2001;37(1 Suppl 1):S65–S136.

17. Diaz-Buxo JA. Chronic peritoneal dialysis prescription In: Daugirdas JT, Ing TS, eds. *Handbook of Dialysis.* 2nd ed. Boston, Mass: Little Brown; 1994:310–327.

18. McCann L, ed. *Pocket Guide to Nutrition Assessment of the Renal Patient.* 3rd ed. New York, NY: National Kidney Foundation; 2002.

Bibliography

Ginsberg N, Fishbane S, Lynn RI. The effect of improved dialytic efficiency on measures of appetite in peritoneal dialysis patients. *J Ren Nutr.* 1996;6:217–221.

Heimbürger O. Residual renal function, peritoneal transport characteristics, and dialysis adequacy in peritoneal dialysis. *Kidney Int.* 1996;50(Suppl 56):S47–S55.

Stover J, ed. *A Clinical Guide to Nutrition Care in End-Stage Renal Disease.* 2nd ed. Chicago, Ill: American Dietetic Association; 1994.

Tattersall JE, Doyle S, Greenwood RN, Farrington K. Kinetic modelling and underdialysis in CAPD patients. *Nephrol Dial Transplant.* 1993;8:535–538.

Tzamaloukas AH. Behind the scenes of the NKF-DOQI guidelines: peritoneal dialysis adequacy. *Dial Transplant.* 1997;26:832–834,853.

Section 17
Volume and Body Surface Area Calculations

Volume Calculations

The following methods may be used to estimate *total body water volume,* or V, in liters. In these formulas, weight (Wt) is measured in kilograms, height (Ht) is measured in centimeters, and age is measured in years. Either of these formulas can be used to determine urea distribution volume for urea kinetic modeling in **peritoneal dialysis patients** (1,2).

Watson Method (3)

Formula 1:

For Men: $V(L) = 2.447 + (0.3362 \times Wt) + (0.1074 \times Ht) - (0.09516 \times Age)$

For Women: $V(L) = -2.097 + (0.2466 \times Wt) + (0.1069 \times Ht)$

Hume-Weyers Method (4)

Formula 2:

For Men: $V(L) = -14.012934 + (0.296785 \times Wt) + (0.194786 \times Ht)$

For Women: $V(L) = -35.270121 + (0.183809 \times Wt) + (0.344547 \times Ht)$

A formula based on bioelectric impedance (BIA) has been developed for use with **hemodialysis patients.** This formula has been shown to correlate better with total body water in hemodialysis patients as measured by BIA than the Watson and Hume-Weyers methods (5). It is recommended as the preferred volume method for urea distribution volume in urea kinetic modeling by the NKF-K/DOQI guidelines (5).

Hemodialysis BIA-Derived Method (6)

Formula 3:

$V(L) = (-0.07493713 \times Age) - (1.01767992 \times Male) + (0.12703384 \times Ht) + (-0.04012056 \times Wt) + (0.57894981 \times Diabetes) - (0.00067247 \times Wt^2) - (0.0348146 \times Age \times Male) + (0.11262857 \times Male \times Wt) + (0.00104135 \times Age \times Wt) + (0.0186104 \times Ht \times Wt)$

Where:

Male = 1 for males, 0 for females
Diabetes = 1 for diabetics, 0 for non-diabetics

Body Surface Area Calculations

The NKF-K/DOQI Clinical Practice Guidelines for Peritoneal Dialysis Adequacy recommend the following equations for calculating body surface area (BSA). These formulas are derived from the general population, but are recommended for use with patients on peritoneal dialysis and should also be acceptable for use with patients on hemodialysis (1). In all formulas, Wt = weight (kg) and Ht = height (cm).

Formula 4: DuBois and DuBois Method (7)

$$BSA (m^2) = 0.007184 \times (Wt^{0.425}) \times (Ht^{0.725})$$

Formula 5: Gehan and George Method (8)

$$BSA (m^2) = 0.0235 \times (Wt^{0.51456}) \times (Ht^{0.42246})$$

Formula 6: Haycock et al Method (9)

$$BSA (m^2) = 0.024265 \times (Wt^{0.5378}) \times (Ht^{0.3964})$$

Adjustment for Amputation

If a patient has an amputation, it must be accounted for in calculating volume and BSA. Table 17.1 lists the percentage of total body weight contributed by certain segments of the body (10). Also listed is the percentage of body surface area (BSA) contributed by the segments of the body (1).

Table 17.1 Percentages of Total Body Weight and Percentages of Body Surface Area Contributed by Segments of the Body

Body Segment	Mean Percentage (%) of Total Body Weight*	Mean Percentage (%) of Body Surface Area†
Entire arm	5.0	10.0
Upper arm (to elbow)	2.7	4.0
Forearm	1.6	3.5
Hand	0.7	2.5
Entire leg	16.0	18.0
Thigh	10.1	8.0
Calf	4.4	6.5
Foot	1.5	3.5

*Reprinted from Osterkamp LK. Current perspective on assessment of human body proportions of relevance to amputees. *J Am Diet Assoc.* 1995; 9:215-218. Reprinted with permission from Elsevier Science (10).

†Reprinted from NKF-K/DOQI clinical practice guidelines for peritoneal dialysis adequacy: update 2000. *Am J Kidney Dis.* 2001;37(1 Suppl 1):S65–S136. Reprinted with permission from the National Kidney Foundation (1).

If several segments are included in the amputation, such as the lower leg consisting of calf and foot, then the percentages are summed to equal the total percentage of the amputation. For example, with a lower leg amputation, the percentages for calf and foot segments would be summed to yield a total amputation weight percentage of 5.9% or total amputation BSA percentage of 10.0%.

Adjusting Volume for Amputation (1)

1. An estimate of full body weight (FBW) is first determined using Formula 7.

$$\textbf{Formula 7:} \text{ Estimated FBW (kg)} = \frac{\text{measured weight}}{[100 - (\% \text{ weight of amputation})]} \times 100$$

2. This weight is then used in the appropriate formula for calculating volume to obtain the estimated volume including the missing limb segments, or the *estimated full body volume.*
3. Divide the full body volume by the full body weight. This yields the proportion of water in 1 kilogram of the patient's weight (number of liters/kg). It is assumed that the proportion of water is the same throughout the entire body.
4. Multiply this proportion by the actual post-amputation weight to determine the *volume adjusted for amputation.*

Example: For a 52–year-old, 5-ft 10-in (178 cm) man weighing 163 lb (74 kg) with a leg amputated to the knee (and receiving peritoneal dialysis):

1. The percentage of total body weight contributed by the missing limb = 1.5 (foot) + 4.4 (calf) = 5.9%

$$\text{Estimated FBW (kg)} = \frac{74}{[100 - 5.9]} \times 100 = \frac{74}{(94.1)} \times 100 = 78.6 \text{ kg}$$

2. Using the Watson Method for volume:

$$V(L) = 2.447 + (0.3362 \times 78.6) + (0.1074 \times 178) - (0.09516 \times 52) = 43.0 \text{ L}$$

3. Proportion of water per kg $= \dfrac{43.0}{78.6} = 0.55$ L/kg
4. Volume adjusted for amputation = $(0.55) \times (74) = 40.7$ L

Adjusting Body Surface Area for Amputation (1)

1. An estimate of full body weight is first determined using Formula 7.
2. This weight is then used in the appropriate formula for calculating BSA to obtain the estimated BSA including the missing limb segments, or the *estimated full BSA.*
3. Determine the percentage BSA contributed by the missing limb segments from the table.
4. To obtain the *BSA adjusted for amputation,* multiply the full BSA times [100 – (%BSA of amputation)], then divide the result by 100.

Example: Using the same individual in the previous example
1. The percentage of total body weight contributed by the missing limb = 1.5 (foot) + 4.4 (calf) = 5.9%

$$\text{Estimated FBW (kg)} = \frac{74}{[100 - 5.9]} \times 100 = \frac{74}{(94.1)} \times 100 = 78.6 \text{ kg}$$

2. Using the DuBois and DuBois method for body surface area:

$$\text{BSA (m}^2) = 0.007184 \times (78.6)^{0.425} \times (178)^{0.725} = 0.007184 \times (6.39) \times (42.81) = 1.97 \text{ m}^2$$

3. The percentage of BSA contributed by the missing limb = 3.5 (foot) + 6.5 (calf) = 10%

4. BSA adjusted for amputation $= \dfrac{1.97 \times [100 - (10)]}{100} = \dfrac{1.97 \times 90}{100} = 1.77 \text{ m}^2$

References

1. NKF-K/DOQI clinical practice guidelines for peritoneal dialysis adequacy: update 2000. *Am J Kidney Dis.* 2001;37(1 Suppl 1):S65–S136.

2. Tzamaloukas AH, Murata GH, Malhotra D, Sena P, Patron A. Urea kinetic modeling in continuous peritoneal dialysis patients: effect of body composition on the methods for estimating urea volume of distribution. *ASAIO J.* 1993;39:M359–M362.

3. Watson PE, Watson ID, Batt RD. Total body water volumes for adult males and females estimated from simple anthropometric measurements. *Am J Clin Nutr.* 1980;33:27–39.

4. Hume R, Weyers E. Relationship between total body water and surface area in normal and obese subjects. *J Clin Pathol.* 1971;24:234–238.

5. NKF-K/DOQI clinical practice guidelines for hemodialysis adequacy: update 2000. *Am J Kidney Dis.* 2001;37(1 Suppl 1):S7–S64.

6. Chertow GM, Lowrie EG, Lew NL, Lazarus JM. Development of a population-specific regression equation to estimate total body water in hemodialysis patients. *Kidney Int.* 1997;51:1578–1582.

7. DuBois D, DuBois EF. A formula to estimate the approximate surface area if height and weight be known. *Nutrition.* 1989;5:303–311.

8. Gehan E, George SL. Estimation of human body surface area from height and weight. *Cancer Chemother Rep.* 1970;54:225–235.

9. Haycock GB, Chir B, Schwartz GJ, Wisotsky DH. Geometric method for measuring body surface area: a height-weight formula validated in infants, children, and adults. *J Pediatr.* 1978;93:62–66.

10. Osterkamp LK. Current perspective on assessment of human body proportions of relevance to amputees. *J Am Diet Assoc.* 1995;95:215–218.

Section 18
Cardiovascular Disease

Cardiovascular disease (CVD) is the leading cause of death in patients with chronic kidney disease (CKD), accounting for approximately 40% of all deaths in the US dialysis population (1). Even after stratification by age, gender, race, and presence of diabetes, the mortality rate from CVD in dialysis patients remains 10 to 20 times higher than the CVD mortality rate in the general population (1–3). In transplant patients, the mortality rate due to CVD is less than that for dialysis patients, but is still about twice that for the general population (1,2).

Patients with CKD are subject to the same risk factors for CVD as the general population, with additional risk factors due to renal disease. Some of these risk factors cannot be modified, such as age and gender. Those that are modifiable include hypertension, lipid abnormalities, hyperglycemia, tobacco use, physical inactivity, elevated homocysteine levels, and calcium/phosphorus/PTH imbalances (1,4).

The American Heart Association (AHA) and the National Heart, Lung, and Blood Institute (NHLBI) of the National Institutes of Health (NIH) have published guidelines for treatment and prevention of CVD in the general population, targeting modifiable risk factors. These guidelines include the AHA Guide to Primary Prevention of Cardiovascular Diseases; the AHA Dietary Guidelines; NHLBI's Sixth Joint National Committee on the Prevention, Detection, Evaluation, and Treatment of High Blood Pressure (JNC VI); and the NHLBI's Third Report of the National Cholesterol Education Program (NCEP) Expert Panel on Detection, Evaluation, and Treatment of High Blood Cholesterol in Adults [Adult Treatment Panel III (ATP III)]. In 1997 a task force was convened by the National Kidney Foundation (NKF) to consider whether strategies for prevention and treatment of CVD in the general population were applicable to patients with CKD (5). The Task Force developed guidelines for prevention and treatment of CVD in CKD and recommended that the risk factors for the general population as well as risk factors specific to renal disease be targeted.

The following is a summary of the risk factors for CVD in CKD and the recommendations made by the NKF Task Force and other national agencies for the areas in which dietitians have an impact. For the complete NKF Task Force executive summary, see reference 5; a brief summary of methods and recommendations is presented in reference 6.

Hypertension

High blood pressure is a major risk factor for CVD in the general population, with studies showing a clear relationship between higher blood pressure levels and higher rates of coronary heart disease, stroke, and heart failure (7). Additionally, in the general population, lowering blood pressure has been shown to reduce the risk of developing or dying from CVD (4,7,8). High blood pressure is also a major risk factor for CVD in patients with CKD, with blood pressure levels tending to increase as renal function deteriorates (4,9,10). Estimates of the prevalence of hypertension in CKD are about 60% to 90% in CKD (predialysis) patients, 75% to 80% in dialysis patients, and 70% to 85% in transplant recipients (1,9,10).

According to the NKF Task Force, the preferred therapy for hypertension is control of extracellular fluid (ECF) volume and maintenance of dry weight through dietary sodium reduction in all CKD populations, diuretics in CKD (predialysis) patients and transplant recipients, and reduction in fluid intake and ultra-filtration in hemodiaysis and peritoneal dialysis patients (10). Because ECF volume control is often not as useful as in the general population, antihypertensive agents may also be necessary to control of ECF volume in CKD patients (10).

Within the general population, additional lifestyle changes are encouraged to reduce blood pressure levels. The JNC VI and the AHA recommend weight control, physical activity, and moderation in alcohol use as measures for prevention and treatment of hypertension (11–13). These lifestyle changes may also benefit CKD patients. In the Modification of Diet in Renal Disease (MDRD) study, weight reductions improved blood pressure in hypertensive CKD (predialysis) patients (14).

Hyperlipidemia

Research has shown that increased total cholesterol and low density lipoprotein cholesterol (LDL-C) levels correlate with risk of CVD in the general population and that reductions in LDL-C levels are associated with decreased risk for CVD (8,13,15). Additionally, a low high-density lipoprotein cholesterol (HDL-C) level is strongly associated with increased risk of CVD (8,15). There is a high prevalence of lipid abnormalities in patients with CKD, with the type and severity of the lipid abnormalities varying depending on the level of renal function, the cause of renal disease, and the type of treatment for renal disease (4,9,16).

The NKF Task Force recommends that virtually every patient with renal disease be screened for hyperlipidemia, and that the NCEP Adult Treatment Panel II guidelines be used for initial classification, treatment initiation, and target cholesterol levels for diet or drug therapy (5,16). Since the publication of the NKF Task Force report, the NCEP released an updated version of the Adult Treatment Panel Guidelines, ATP III, with more emphasis on LDL-C. It is reasonable to assume that these modifications to the NCEP guidelines would also be relevant to the CKD population. The NKF Task Force recommendations, modified to include changes to the ATP guidelines, are as follows:

- In adults aged 20 years or older, a fasting lipoprotein profile (total cholesterol, LDL-C, HDL-C, and triglyceride) should be obtained every 5 years (15). If the testing opportunity is nonfasting, only total cholesterol and HDL-C will be usable (15). If this is the case, a follow-up lipoprotein profile is recommended if total cholesterol is 200 mg/dL or more or HDL-C is less than 40 mg/dL (15).
- Patients with CKD should be considered the highest risk group (coronary heart disease [CHD] and CHD risk equivalents) (16). For patients in the highest risk group, LDL-C goal is less than 100 mg/dL (15). Therapeutic lifestyle changes (TLC) are recommended for LDL-C of 100 mg/dL or more, and drug therapy should be considered for LDL-C of 130 mg/dL or more (15). TLC includes a diet low in cholesterol and saturated fat, weight management, and increased physical activity.
- TLC is recommended for patients with CKD, but most patients with hyperlipidemia also require drug therapy (16).
- Elevated serum triglyceride or low HDL-C levels, with or without increased LDL-C levels, should be treated with TLC (15). The value of drug therapy to reduce CVD risk is uncertain (16).

More information about the NCEP ATP III guidelines can be found in reference 15. The complete NKF Task Force guidelines for hyperlipidemia in patients with CKD is available in reference 16.

Hyperglycemia

Diabetes has been shown to be an independent risk factor for CVD in the general population and in patients with CKD (5,17). It has also been suggested that hyperglycemia itself may be a risk factor for

CVD, although it is not clear if improved control of hyperglycemia in diabetic patients reduces the risk of CVD (8). Hyperglycemia may affect atherogenesis by causing endothelial injury, affecting plaque formation through LDL glycation, enhancing platelet aggregation, increasing platelet generation of vasoconstrictor prostanoids, and inducing a procoagulant state (18). In addition to hyperglycemia, patients with diabetes often have other risk factors that increase the likelihood of development of CVD (8). In particular, type 2 diabetes is commonly associated with the metabolic syndrome, a group of risk factors for CVD including dyslipidemia, hypertension, and enhancement of prothrombotic factors (13,17). Insulin resistance is closely tied to the metabolic syndrome as well, and also seems to predispose patients for the development of CVD (17).

The NKF Task Force recommends intensive glycemic control in CKD (predialysis) patients (specifically patients with microalbuminuria caused by diabetic renal disease) and in transplant recipients (18). For these patient populations, the Task Force suggests following the American Diabetes Association's recommendations and reducing blood glucose levels to normal or near normal in most patients with type 1 or type 2 diabetes (18). Glycemic control may slow the progression or development of diabetic renal disease in CKD (predialysis) and transplant patients, reduce the danger of metabolic and infectious complications from uncontrolled hyperglycemia, and improve hyperlipidemia (18). Improved control of hyperglycemia may possibly decrease the risk of CVD as well. In patients on dialysis, the achievement of intensive glycemic controls needs to be determined on an individual basis (18). Because damage to the kidneys has already occurred and cannot be reversed with intensive glycemic control, the advantage of achieving intense control over glycemic levels must be balanced against the difficulty for the patient to maintain a renal and diabetic diet and the risk for decreasing nutritional status with a more restrictive diet.

Tobacco Use

Cigarette smoking is a strong risk factor for CVD, with as many as 30% of all coronary heart disease deaths in the United States attributable to smoking (19). Additionally, risk of CVD decreases rapidly with cessation of smoking (8,19). In patients with CKD, smoking has also been shown to be an independent risk factor for CVD (9,20). Smoking affects normal kidney function both directly and indirectly, and is associated with progression of renal failure in diabetics (20).

The effect of smoking cessation on renal outcomes is unknown (20), but based on the effect seen in the general population, the NKF Task Force considers it reasonable to expect that smoking cessation will improve CVD outcomes in patients with CKD (20). The Task Force recommends using general population guidelines for counseling and nicotine replacement for patients with CKD (20). "Treating Tobacco Use and Dependence" is a clinical practice guideline, published by the US Department of Health and Human Services, that contains strategies and recommendations to assist clinicians in delivering and supporting effective treatments for tobacco use and dependence (21). Brief clinical interventions that can be easily delivered in the primary care setting and intensive clinical interventions appropriate for tobacco dependence treatment specialists are provided in the guideline (21). Recommendations for use of pharmacotherapies are also presented (21). The AHA has also issued an advisory for health care professionals, emphasizing the value of smoking cessation and outlining intervention guidelines found to be helpful in promoting smoking cessation and recommendations for nicotine patch replacement therapy (19).

Physical Inactivity

Lack of physical activity is recognized as a risk factor for coronary artery disease (22,23). Increasing physical activity reduces mortality from CVD and also favorably modifies other CVD risk factors, including hypertension, insulin resistance, hyperlipidemia, and obesity (22–24).

Recommendations for increased physical activity in the general population have been developed by the AHA and NIH, among others (22,24). These guidelines recommend 30 minutes of moderate intensity exercise on most or all days of the week (20,22–24). This may include short periods of moderate intensity activity (at least 10 minutes) with an accumulated duration of at least 30 minutes on most days (22,24). The NKF Task Force states that the normal level of physical activity is reduced among patients with CKD, but the recommended level of moderate physical activity is feasible in many patients with CKD and should be encouraged (5,20). Physical activity can be increased through counseling and exercise training (20).

The importance of physical activity among the CKD population has also been emphasized in terms of patient rehabilitation. Section 19 reviews the role of exercise in rehabilitation and provides resources for encouraging increased physical activity in patients with CKD.

Homocysteine

Homocysteine is a sulfur-containing amino acid that is formed during the metabolism of methionine. There is considerable evidence that an association exists between hyperhomocysteinemia and CVD and that an increase in homocysteine levels could increase risk for CVD (13,25). Not all studies have confirmed this association, however (13,25). For the general population, the AHA suggests that fasting homocysteine levels be checked in "high-risk" patients, such as those with a strong family history of premature atherosclerosis or with arterial occlusive diseases as well as members of their families (25). Subjects with impaired renal function are also considered "high-risk" (25). Homocysteine levels are elevated in patients with CKD and are approximately twice as high in dialysis and transplant patients compared with the general population (4,26). As in the general population, there is strong evidence for an association between homocysteine levels and CVD in CKD patients, although the evidence is not conclusive and no data yet exist demonstrating that lowering homocysteine levels will reduce risk for CVD (1,4,26,27). However, treatment of hyperhomocysteinemia is generally safe and relatively inexpensive (4,20). Supplementation with high-dose folic acid alone or in combination with vitamin B-12 or B-6 can reduce homocysteine levels by 25% to 30% in CKD patients (20,26,27).

Based on study results, the NKF Task Force recommends 5 mg/day of folic acid in combination with 0.4 mg/day vitamin B-12 and 50 mg/day vitamin B-6 for reducing homocysteine levels (20). The optimal doses and combinations of these vitamins have yet to be determined, though, and even a reduction of 30% results in normal homocysteine levels in only a minority of dialysis patients with elevated homocysteine levels (1,4).

Cardiovascular Calicification

Calcification of cardiac tissues frequently occurs in patients receiving dialysis. Studies using either echocardiography or electron-beam computed tomography have shown cardiovascular calcification in 45% to 59% of current dialysis patients, and calcification has been reported on autopsy in up to 60% of patients who had undergone dialysis (28–32). The calcium deposits have been found in various cardiac tissues and structures, including the myocardium, pericardium, conduction system, aortic and mitral valves, small myocardial arteries, and coronary arteries (29,31–34). Such calcification can damage normal cardiac tissues and contribute to mitral and aortic valve stenosis and insufficiency, abnormal conduction and arrhythmia, myocardial ischemia, left ventricular dysfunction, complete heart block, and congestive heart failure (29,31,32). Several factors are associated with cardiac calcification, including hyperphosphatemia, elevated calcium-phosphorus product (Ca x P), excess calcium intake, elevated levels of parathyroid hormone (PTH), older age, and increased dialysis duration (29,31–34).

Phosphorus

Hyperphosphatemia is prevalent in the dialysis population and is associated with an increased mortality rate. In a retrospective study of 6,407 patients receiving dialysis, those with serum phosphorus levels more than 6.5 mg/dL had a 27% greater risk of death than those patients with phosphorus levels in the range of 2.4 to 6.5 mg/dL (29,35). A follow-up study to this study found a 56% increase in risk of death from coronary artery disease in those patients with serum phosphorus more than 6.5 mg/dL and an 11% increase in mortality risk for each 1 mg/dL increase in phosphorus (28,29,36). The risk for sudden death also increased 27% for those with phosphorus levels more than 6.5 mg/dL (28,36). This increased mortality risk may be due in part to cardiovascular calcification. Hyperphosphatemia has been directly associated with coronary artery calcification and also contributes to elevated Ca x P and hyperparathyroidism, two other factors associated with cardiovascular calcification (28,34,37,38).

Calcium-Phosphorus Product (Ca x P)

Several studies have shown an association between Ca x P and cardiovascular calcification. In one study of 92 chronic hemodialysis patients, patients with mitral valve calcification had significantly higher maximum Ca x P than those without calcification (31). The highest mean Ca x P in 6 successive months was also calculated and found to be significantly higher in patients with mitral valve calcification (31). In a second study of 39 young patients undergoing dialysis, Ca x P was strongly associated with coronary artery calcification with the mean Ca x P over 6 months significantly higher in the patients with coronary artery calcification than in those without evidence of calcification (34). Other studies have found similar results, with cardiovascular calcification occurring at Ca x P levels between 55 to 65, much less than the standard target level of 70 to 75 (28,29,31). Ca x P levels more than 72 have even been linked to increased risk of death (35). Overall mortality risk was shown to be 34% greater in patients with Ca x P more than 72 relative to those with Ca x P between 42 and 52 (35). Risk of death due to sudden death was also increased in those with elevated Ca x P levels (36).

Calcium Intake

Many dialysis patients receive high levels of calcium from use of calcium-based phosphate binders and influx of calcium from the dialysate bath (28,39). Use of vitamin D therapy to control PTH can enhance gastrointestinal uptake of calcium as well (28). A high calcium burden can lead to increased serum calcium levels and elevated Ca x P, thus contributing to the development of cardiovascular calcification (38,39). Vascular calcification has been associated directly with calcium intake even when calcium and Ca x P levels have not been elevated (33,34). Dose of calcium carbonate prescribed was significantly associated with arterial calcification in a group of 120 dialysis patients in spite of mean calcium levels ranging from 9.2 to 10.4 mg/dL and mean Ca x P ranging from 50.9 to 57.1 (33). In a study of 39 young dialysis patients, those found to have coronary artery calcification were prescribed a significantly higher dose of oral calcium (6,456 ± 4,278 mg/day) than those with no calcification (3,325 ± 1,490 mg/day), but mean serum calcium levels remained within acceptable limits and were not associated with calcification (34).

Parathyroid Hormone (PTH)

Secondary hyperparathyroidism in dialysis patients has been linked to the development of soft tissue calcification (28,32,37). With elevated PTH levels, bone resorption is increased, facilitating the release of calcium and phosphorus from the bone and promoting elevations in serum calcium, phosphorus, and/or Ca x P levels (37). Additionally, chronically elevated PTH levels can result in the accumulation of calcium within cells' mitochondria (28). When excess calcium has entered the cell, calcification can occur within the mitochondria, which then serves as a nucleus for proliferation of the calcification within and outside the cell (28). Excess PTH also can affect cardiovascular structure and function in ways other than through tissue calcification. Hyperparathyroidism has been linked with left ventricular hypertrophy and increased left ventricular mass, glucose intolerance and insulin resistance, hypertension, lipid disturbances, and atherosclerosis (28,32).

Low PTH levels resulting in adynamic bone disease may also affect the development of cardiovascular calcification. Patients with adynamic bone disease or low bone turnover are more likely to develop hypercalcemia due to the bone's decreased capacity to buffer calcium (28,33,40). Hyperphosphatemia can similarly occur with low bone activity (33). In patients with elevated phosphorus levels, doses of phosphate binders are often higher, and if calcium-based binders are used, calcium intake will be increased.

Recommendations

Recommendations for calcium, phosphorus, and PTH management have been made to address the high prevalence of cardiovascular calcification in the dialysis population. Recently, Block and Port have recommended maintaining phosphorus levels between 2.5 and 5.5 mg/dL, calcium levels between 9.2 and 9.6 mg/dL, and Ca x P less than 55, with optimal levels being as close to normal serum values as can be achieved (28,40). Other authors have suggested even lower levels, with phosphorus levels to be kept less than 5.0 mg/dL and Ca x P less than 50 to 55 (41,42). The recommended range for PTH levels generally lies between 100 to 300 pg/mL (28,43–46). To maintain these levels and avoid excess calcium intake, use of non–calcium-containing phosphate binders and vitamin D analogs may prove beneficial (28).

CKD (predialysis) and Transplantation

Little information is available in the scientific literature about cardiovascular calcification in CKD (predialysis) or transplantation. However, calcium, phosphorus, and PTH imbalances are known to develop in the early stages of CKD, so it is not without reason to suspect that the risk of calcification may be increased in this population as well. Limiting phosphorus intake early in CKD may help prevent elevation of PTH (47). Maintenance of serum calcium and phosphorus levels as close to normal as possible may help to decrease potential for the development of cardiovascular calcification in CKD (predialysis) and transplant recipients.

References

1. Sarnak MJ, Levey AS. Cardiovascular disease and chronic renal disease: a new paradigm. *Am J Kidney Dis*. 2000;35(4 Suppl 1):S117–S131.

2. Foley RN, Parfrey PS, Sarnak MJ. Epidemiology of cardiovascular disease in chronic renal disease. *J Am Soc Nephrol*. 1998;9:S16–S23.

3. Foley RN, Parfrey PS, Sarnak MJ. Cardiovascular disease in chronic renal disease: clinical epidemiology of cardiovascular disease in chronic renal disease. *Am J Kidney Dis*. 1998;32 (5 Suppl 3):S112–S119.

4. Coresh J, Longenecker JC, Miller ER, Young HJ, Klag MJ. Epidemiology of cardiovascular risk factors in chronic renal disease. *J Am Soc Nephrol*. 1998;9:S24–S30.

5. Levey AS. Executive summary: controlling the epidemic of cardiovascular disease in chronic renal disease: where do we start? *Am J Kidney Dis*. 1998;32 (5 Suppl 3):S5–S13.

6. Meyer KB, Levey AS. Controlling the epidemic of cardiovascular disease in chronic renal disease: report from the National Kidney Foundation Task Force on Cardiovascular Disease. *J Am Soc Nephrol*. 1998;9:S31–S42.

7. Chobanian AV, Hill M. National Heart, Lung and Blood Institute Workshop on Sodium and Blood Pressure: a critical review of current scientific evidence. *Hypertension*. 2000;35:858–863.

8. Grundy SM, Balady GJ, Criqui MH, Fletcher G, Greenland P, Hiratzka LF, Houston-Miller N, Kris-Etherton P, Krumholz HM, LaRosa J, Ockene IS, Pearson TA, Reed J, Washington R, Smith SC. Primary prevention of coronary heart disease: guidance from Framingham: a statement for healthcare professionals from the AHA Task Force on Risk Reduction. *Circulation*. 1998;97:1876–1887.

9. Wheeler DC. Cardiovascular risk factors in patients with chronic renal failure. *J Ren Nutr*. 1997;7:182–186.

10. Milloux LU, Levey AS. Hypertension in patients with chronic renal disease. *Am J Kidney Dis*. 1998;32(5 Suppl 3):S120–S141.

11. The sixth report of the Joint National Committee on Prevention, Detection, Evaluation, and Treatment of High Blood Pressure. *Arch Intern Med.* 1997;157:2413–2446.

12. Grundy SM, Balady GJ, Criqui MH, Fletcher G, Greenland P, Hiratzka LF, Houston-Miller N, Kris-Etherton P, Krumholz HM, LaRosa J, Ockene IS, Pearson TA, Reed J, Washington R, Smith SC. Guide to primary prevention of cardiovascular diseases: a statement for healthcare professionals from the Task Force on Risk Reduction. *Circulation.* 1997;95:2329–2331.

13. Krauss RM, Eckel RH, Howard B, Appel LJ, Daniels SR, Deckelbaum RJ, Erdman JW, Kris-Etherton P, Goldberg IJ, Kotchen TA, Lichtenstein AH, Mitch WE, Mullis R, Robinson K, Wylie-Rosett J, St Jeor S, Suttie J, Tribble DL, Bazzarre TL. AHA dietary guidelines: revision 2000: a statement for healthcare professionals from the Nutrition Committee of the American Heart Association. *Circulation.* 2000;102:2284–2299.

14. Yamamoto ME, Olson MB, Fine J, Powers S, Stollar C. The effect of sodium restriction and weight reduction on blood pressure of patients with hypertension and chronic renal disease. *J Ren Nutr.* 1997;7:25–32.

15. National Cholesterol Education Program. Executive summary of the third report of the National Cholesterol Education Program (NCEP) Expert Panel on Detection, Evaluation, and Treatment of High Blood Cholesterol in Adults (Adult Treatment Panel III). *JAMA.* 2001;285:2486–2497.

16. Kasiske BL. Hyperlipidemia in patients with chronic renal disease. *Am J Kidney Dis.* 1998;32(5 Suppl 3):S142–S156.

17. Grundy SM, Benjamin IJ, Burke GL, Chait A, Eckel RH, Howard BV, Mitch W, Smith SC, Sowers JR. Diabetes and cardiovascular disease: a statement for healthcare professionals from the American Heart Association. *Circulation.* 1999;100:1134–1146.

18. Manske CL. Hyperglycemia and intensive glycemic control in diabetic patients with chronic renal disease. *Am J Kidney Dis.* 1998;32(5 Suppl 3):S157–S171.

19. Ockene IS, Houston Miller N. Cigarette smoking, cardiovascular disease, and stroke: a statement for healthcare professionals from the American Heart Association. *Circulation.* 1997;96:3243–3247.

20. Beto JA, Bansal VK. Interventions for other risk factors: tobacco use, physical inactivity, menopause, and homocysteine. *Am J Kidney Dis.* 1998;32(Suppl 3):S172–S184.

21. Fiore MC, Bailey WC, Cohen SJ, Dorfman SF, Goldstein MG, Gritz ER, Heyman RB, Jaen CR, Kottke TE, Lando HA, Mecklenburg RE, Mullen PD, Nett LM, Robinson L, Stitzer ML, Tommasello AC, Villejo L, Wewers ME. *Treating Tobacco Use and Dependence. Clinical Practice Guideline.* Rockville, Md: US Department of Health and Human Services, Public Health Service; 2000.

22. Fletcher GF, Balady G, Blair SN, Blumenthal J, Caspersen C, Chaitman B, Epstein S, Sivarajan Froelicher ES, Froelicher VF, Pina IL, Pollock ML. Statement on exercise: benefits and recommendations for physical activity programs for all Americans: a statement for health professionals by the Committee on Exercise and Cardiac Rehabilitation of the Council on Clinical Cardiology, American Heart Association. *Circulation.* 1996;94:857–862.

23. Wenger NK. Lipid metabolism, physical activity, and postmenopausal hormone therapy. *Am J Kidney Dis.* 1998;32(5 Suppl 3):S80–S88.

24. Physical Activity and Cardiovascular Health. NIH Consensus Statement Online. December 18–20, 1995. 13(3):1–33. Available at: http://consensus.nih.gov/cons/101/101_statement.htm. Accessed March 23, 2002.

25. Malinow MR, Bostom AG, Krauss RM. Homocysteine, diet, and cardiovascular diseases: a statement for healthcare professionals from the Nutrition Committee, American Heart Association. *Circulation.* 1999;99:178–182.

26. Kronenberg F. Homocysteine, lipoprotein(a), and fibrinogen: metabolic risk factors for cardiovascular complications of renal disease. *Curr Opin Nephrol Hypertens.* 1998;7:271–278.

27. Bostom AG, Culleton BF. Hyperhomocysteinemia in chronic renal disease. *J Am Soc Nephrol.* 1999;10:891–900.

28. Block GA, Port FK. Re-evaluation of risks associated with hyperphosphatemia and hyperparathyroidism in dialysis patients: recommendations for a change in management. *Am J Kidney Dis.* 2000;35:1226–1237.

29. Llach F. Cardiac calcification: dealing with another risk factor in patients with kidney failure. *Semin Dial.* 1999;12:293–295.

30. Braun J, Oldendorf M, Moshage W, Heidler R, Zeitler E, Luft FC. Electron beam computed tomography in the evaluation of cardiac calcifications in chronic dialysis patients. *Am J Kidney Dis*. 1996;27:394–401.

31. Ribeiro S, Ramos A, Brandao A, Rebelo JR, Guerra A, Resina C, Vila-Lobos A, Carvalho F, Remedio F, Ribeiro F. Cardiac valve calcification in haemodialysis patients: role of calcium-phosphate metabolism. *Nephrol Dial Transplant*. 1998;13:2037–2040.

32. Rostand SG, Drueke TB. Parathyroid hormone, vitamin D, and cardiovascular disease in chronic renal failure. *Kidney Int*. 1999;56:383–392.

33. Guerin AP, London GM, Marchais SJ, Metivier F. Arterial stiffening and vascular calcifications in end-stage renal disease. *Nephrol Dial Transplant*. 2000;15:1014–1021.

34. Goodman WG, Goldin J, Kuizon BD, Yoon C, Gales B, Sider D, Wang Y, Chung J, Emerick A, Greaser L, Elashoff RM, Salusky IB. Coronary-artery calcification in young adults with end-stage renal disease who are undergoing dialysis. *N Engl J Med* 2000;342:1478–1483.

35. Block GA, Hulbert-Shearon TE, Levin NW, Port FK. Association of serum phosphorus and calcium x phosphate product with mortality risk in chronic hemodialysis patients: a national study. *Am J Kidney Dis*. 1998;31:607–617.

36. Levin NW, Hulbert-Shearon TE, Strawderman RL, Port FK. Which causes of death are related to hyperphosphatemia in hemodialysis patients? Presented at: 8th Annual National Kidney Foundation Clinical Nephrology Meetings, Washington, DC, May 1, 1999.

37. Llach F, Yudd M. Pathogenic, clinical, and therapeutic aspects of secondary hyperparathyroidism in chronic renal failure. *Am J Kidney Dis*. 1998;32(4 Suppl 2):S3–S12.

38. Slatopolsky E, Brown A, Dusso A. role of phosphorus in the pathogenesis of secondary hyperparathyroidism. *Am J Kidney Dis*. 2001;37(1 Suppl 2):S54–S57.

39. Raggi P. Imaging of cardiovascular calcifications with electron beam tomography in hemodialysis patients. *Am J Kidney Dis*. 2001;37(1 Suppl 2):S62–S65.

40. Block GA. Reevaluating the risks of secondary hyperparathyroidism and hyperphosphatemia. Presented at: Northwest Renal Dietitians Annual Meeting, Portland, Ore, March 7, 2000.

41. Malluche HH, Monier-Faugere MC. Understanding and managing hyperphosphatemia in patients with chronic renal disease. *Clin Nephrol*. 1999;52:267–277.

42. Cannata-Andia JB, Rodriguez-Garcia, M. Hyperphosphataemia as a cardiovascular risk factor—how to manage the problem. *Nephrol Dial Transplant*. 2002;17(Suppl 11):16–19.

43. Wang M, Hercz G, Sherrard DJ, Maloney NA, Segre GV, Pei Y. Relationship between intact 1–84 parathyroid hormone and bone histomorphometric parameters in dialysis patients without aluminum toxicity. *Am J Kidney Dis*. 1995;26:836–844.

44. Goodman WG, Jüppner H, Salusky IB, Sherrard DJ. Parathyroid hormone (PTH), PTH-derived peptides, and new PTH assays in renal osteodystrophy. *Kidney Int*. 2003;63:1–11.

45. Ho LT, Sprague SM. Renal osteodystrophy in chronic renal failure. *Semin Nephrol*. 2002;22:488–493.

46. Avram MM. Risks and monitoring of elevated parathyroid hormone in chronic renal failure (a review). *Dial Transplant*. 2001;30:147–155.

47. Kates DM, Sherrard D, Andress DL. Evidence that serum phosphate is independently associated with serum PTH in patients with chronic renal failure. *Am J Kidney Dis*. 1997;30:809–813.

Section 19
Exercise and Rehabilitation

Advances in medical technology and pharmacology have made treatment for kidney failure more effective, allowing patients to achieve an improved quality of life with the help of rehabilitation efforts. The Life Options Rehabilitation Advisory Council (LORAC), an interdisciplinary council comprised of patients and their family members, providers, government representatives, researchers, and private business individuals, was formed out of the realization that renal rehabilitation had not yet been adequately addressed on a national scale despite the improved potential for rehabilitation of patients with chronic kidney disease (CKD). LORAC released a report in 1994 defining rehabilitation as "a coordinated program of medical treatment, education, counseling, dietary, and exercise regimens designed to maximize the vocational potential, functional status, and quality of life of dialysis patients" (1). The main outcome goals identified by LORAC include (1):

- Employment for those who are able to work, including patients older than 65 years who wish to work
- Enhanced fitness to improve physical functioning for all patients
- Improved understanding about adaptation and the options for living well with dialysis
- Increased control over the effects of kidney disease and dialysis
- Resumption of activities enjoyed prior to dialysis

Achieving and maintaining normal nutritional status is critical for successful rehabilitation. Malnutrition and wasting directly affect functional capacity, particularly muscle function and quality of life, leading to poor prognosis and impaired rehabilitation (2,3). As part of the dialysis team, the dietitian's role is essential for achieving each of the goals set by LORAC.

Five core areas, termed the "Five Es," were identified by LORAC as fundamental in the rehabilitation of CKD patients: encouragement, education, exercise, employment, and evaluation (4). Dietitians can contribute to rehabilitation in several core areas. In particular, exercise is an area in which dietitians can play a key role. Nutritional status impacts exercise capacity and the ability of a patient to achieve a certain level of functional ability (3). Conversely, physical activity has been shown to have a positive effect on protein utilization and retention, and may help to counteract the wasting syndrome commonly seen in CKD (predialysis and dialysis) patients (2,3). Exercise can also improve blood pressure control, lipid metabolism, glucose tolerance, insulin sensitivity, and hematocrit levels in CKD patients, including transplant patients, and may reduce the risk of osteoporosis (3,5–7). Additional benefits include weight control, maintenance of muscle mass, and enhanced physical ability, which can allow patients to participate in the activities that they enjoy and will ultimately contribute to an increased quality of life (7–9). Dietitians can support patient rehabilitation in this area by educating the patient about the importance of nutrition in exercise and maintenance of functional ability and by promoting positive nutritional practices to maintain good nutritional status. Encouraging patients to participate in routine exercise and actively participating in the development of exercise programs within the renal community are additional ways in which dietitians can help promote patient rehabilitation.

Resources are available to assist patients in starting an exercise program and help health care staff develop and implement exercise programs for patients. LORAC, through help from Amgen, has published a guide for patients entitled *Exercise: A Guide for People on Dialysis* as part of a comprehensive program for patients and health care staff designed to encourage exercise in the dialysis population (10). Also available from LORAC are 3 booklets for health professionals: *Exercise for the Dialysis Patient: A Guide for the Nephrologist; Exercise for the Dialysis Patient: A Prescribing Guide;* and *Exercise for the Dialysis Patient: A Guide for the Dialysis Team.* These guides are accessible through the LORAC Web site (listed later in this section). LORAC also publishes the *Renal Rehabilitation Report* in cooperation with *Nephrology News & Issues* on a quarterly basis. This newsletter for dialysis professionals and patients highlights various aspects of rehabilitation, including effective programs and projects and ideas for research. Copies of the *Renal Rehabilitation Report* can be accessed through the LORAC Web site. Kidney School, an interactive, internet-based program to teach people about kidney disease and its treatment, is maintained by LORAC and contains a module titled "Staying Active with Kidney Disease." An entire issue of *Advances in Renal Replacement Therapy* has been dedicated to the topic of exercise and includes articles discussing the decreased physical functioning in dialysis patients, importance of exercise in improving physical functioning, and steps the renal community can take to help patients improve physical status (11). The President's Council on Physical Fitness and Sports offers a patient-oriented exercise guide, *Pep Up Your Life: A Fitness Book for Mid-Life and Older Persons,* which focuses on improving strength, flexibility, and endurance for older patients and those with reduced exercise tolerance (12). This and additional information can be obtained from the following resources:

Exercise: A Guide for People on Dialysis
Exercise for the Dialysis Patient: A Guide for the Dialysis Team
Exercise for the Dialysis Patient: A Guide for the Nephrologist
Exercise for the Dialysis Patient: A Prescribing Guide
Renal Rehabilitation Report Newsletter
The Life Options Rehabilitation Program (LORAC)
603 Science Dr
Madison, WI 53711-1074
800/468-7777
E-mail: lifeoptions@medmed.com
http://www.lifeoptions.org
http://www.kidneyschool.org

Pep Up Your Life: A Fitness Book for Mid-Life and Older Persons
The President's Council on Physical Fitness and Sports
http://www.fitness.gov/activelife/activelife.html

Staying Fit with Kidney Disease (brochure #05-02)
National Kidney Foundation, Inc
30 E 33rd St
New York, NY 10016
800/622-9010
http://www.kidney.org

References

1. The Life Options Rehabilitation Advisory Council. *Renal Rehabilitation: Bridging the Barriers.* Madison, Wis: Medical Education Institute; 1994.

2. Castaneda C. The relationship between rehabilitation and nutrition status in renal disease patients. *Contemp Dial Nephrol.* 1997;18:18–21.

3. Castaneda C, Grossi L, Dwyer J. Potential benefits of resistance exercise training on nutritional status in renal failure. *J Ren Nutr.* 1998;8:2–10.

4. Oberley ET, Sadler JH, Stec P. Renal rehabilitation: obstacles, progress, and prospects for the future. *Am J Kidney Dis.* 2000;35(4 Suppl 1):S141–S147.

5. Fitts S. Physical benefits and challenges of exercise for people with chronic renal disease. *J Ren Nutr.* 1997; 7:123–128.

6. Beto JA, Bansal VK. Interventions for other risk factors: tobacco use, physical inactivity, menopause, and homocysteine. *Am J Kidney Dis.* 1998;32(5 Suppl 3):S172–S184.

7. Wenger NK. Lipid metabolism, physical activity, and postmenopausal hormone therapy. *Am J Kidney Dis.* 1998;32(5 Suppl 3):S80–S88.

8. Carey S, Painter P. An exercise program for CAPD patients. *Nephrol News Issues.* 1997;11:15–16,18.

9. Painter P. The importance of exercise training in rehabilitation of patients with end-stage renal disease. *Am J Kidney Dis.* 1994;24(1 Suppl 1):S2–S9.

10. The Life Options Rehabilitation Advisory Council. *Exercise for the Dialysis Patient: A Comprehensive Program.* Madison, Wis: Medical Education Institute; 1995.

11. Painter P, Johansen K, eds. Physical functioning in end-stage renal disease. *Adv Ren Replace Ther.* 1999; 6(theme issue):107–194.

12. President's Council on Physical Fitness and Sports. Pep Up Your Life: A Fitness Book for Mid-Life and Older Persons. Available at: http://www.fitness.gov/activelife/activelife.html. Accessed May 25, 2003.

Bibliography

Casaburi R. Rehabilitative exercise training in chronic renal failure. In: Kopple J, Massry S, eds. *Nutritional Management of Renal Disease.* Baltimore, Md: Williams & Wilkins; 1997:817–841.

Heacock P, Nabel J, Norton P, Heile S, Royse D. An exploration of the relationship between nutritional status and quality of life in chronic hemodialysis patients. *J Ren Nutr.* 1996;6:152–157.

Kouidi E, Albani M, Natsis K, Megalopoulos A, Gigis P, Guiba-Tziampiri O, Tourkantonis A, Deligiannis A. The effects of exercise training on muscle atrophy in haemodialysis patients. *Nephrol Dial Transplant.* 1998; 13:685–699.

Section 20
Immunosuppressant Drugs and Nutritional Side Effects

Drug	Nutritional Side Effects	Nutrition Plan
Cyclosporine (Neoral)[a] (Sandimmune)[a] (Gengraf)[b]	• Hyperglycemia, glucose intolerance • Hyperlipidemia • Nausea/vomiting • Diarrhea • Anorexia • Mouth sores • Hyperkalemia • Hypomagnesemia • Hypertension • Edema • Fever • Pancreatitis • Increased bone resorption	• Monitor blood sugar, may need to limit carbohydrates. • Reduce fat intake. • Monitor for adequate intake, try antiemetic medications. • Review drugs and consider a substitute for those that may be causing diarrhea, monitor and replace fluids as needed. • Monitor for adequate intake, suggest frequent small meals. • Avoid foods that irritate mouth. • Restrict potassium intake. • Supplement with magnesium-rich foods or supplements. • Restrict sodium intake, maintain a healthy weight, encourage regular exercise. • Restrict sodium intake. • Monitor dietary and fluid intake. • Reduce fat intake, initiate TPN if pancreatitis is severe. • Monitor calcium and phosphorus levels; ensure adequate calcium and vitamin D intake; consider need for calcitonin, hormonal replacement, bisphosphonates; encourage weight-bearing exercise, smoking cessation.
Mycophenolate mofetil (CellCept)[c]	• Hyperglycemia, glucose intolerance • Hypercholesterolemia • Nausea/vomiting • Diarrhea • Anorexia • Abdominal pain • Hyperkalemia • Hypokalemia • Hypomagnesemia • Hypophosphatemia • Hypertension • Edema	• Monitor blood sugar, may need to limit carbohydrates. • Reduce fat and cholesterol intake. • Monitor for adequate intake, try antiemetic medications. • Review drugs and consider a substitute for those that may be causing diarrhea, monitor and replace fluids as needed. • Monitor for adequate intake, suggest frequent small meals. • Monitor for adequate intake. • Restrict potassium intake. • Supplement with potassium-rich foods or supplements. • Supplement with magnesium-rich foods or supplements. • Supplement with phosphorus-rich foods or supplements. • Restrict sodium intake, maintain a healthy weight, encourage regular exercise. • Restrict sodium intake.

continues next page

Drug	Nutritional Side Effects	Nutrition Plan (continued)
Glucocorticoids (prednisone) (Deltasone)[d] (Meticorten)[e] (Orasone)[f] (Sterapred)[g]	• Hyperglycemia, glucose intolerance • Hyperlipidemia • Nausea/vomiting • Protein catabolism, muscle wasting • Impaired wound healing • Hypokalemia • Sodium and fluid retention • Hypertension • Hyperphagia, obesity, weight gain • Increased gastric acid secretion • Pancreatitis • Osteoporosis, increased calcium excretion, decreased calcium absorption from gut, hypophosphatemia	• Monitor blood sugar, may need to limit carbohydrates. • Reduce fat intake. • Monitor for adequate intake, try antiemetic medications. • Ensure adequate protein intake. • Ensure adequate protein intake, consider need for vitamin A or C or zinc. • Supplement with potassium-rich foods or supplements. • Restrict sodium intake. • Restrict sodium intake, maintain a healthy weight, encourage regular exercise. • Behavior modification to avoid overeating, encourage regular exercise, reduce fat and calorie intake. • Avoid gastric irritants. • Reduce fat intake, initiate TPN if pancreatitis is severe. • Monitor calcium and phosphorus levels; ensure adequate calcium and vitamin D intake; consider need for calcitonin, hormonal replacement, bisphosphonates; encourage weight-bearing exercise, smoking cessation.
Azathioprine (Imuran)[h]	• Nausea/vomiting • Diarrhea • Esophagitis, mucositis • Altered taste acuity • Fever • Pancreatitis	• Monitor for adequate intake, try antiemetic medications. • Review drugs and consider a substitute for those that may be causing diarrhea, monitor and replace fluids as needed. • Avoid foods that irritate throat. • Offer a variety of foods with different tastes, consider zinc supplementation. • Monitor dietary and fluid intake. • Reduce fat intake, initiate TPN if pancreatitis is severe.
Anti-thymocyte Globulin (ATG) (Thymoglobulin)[j]	• Nausea/vomiting • Diarrhea • Abdominal pain • Hyperkalemia • Hypertension, edema • Hypotension	• Monitor for adequate intake, try antiemetic medications. • Review drugs and consider a substitute for those that may be causing diarrhea, monitor and replace fluids as needed. • Monitor for adequate intake. • Restrict potassium intake. • Restrict sodium intake. • Maintain adequate fluid status.
Sirolimus (Rapamune)[k]	• Hyperglycemia, glucose intolerance • Hyperlipidemia • Nausea/vomiting • Diarrhea • Anorexia • Hypokalemia • Hypertension, edema	• Monitor blood sugar, may need to limit carbohydrates. • Reduce fat intake. • Monitor for adequate intake, try antiemetic medications. • Review drugs and consider a substitute for those that may be causing diarrhea, monitor and replace fluids as needed. • Monitor for adequate intake, suggest frequent small meals. • Supplement with potassium-rich foods or supplements. • Restrict sodium intake.

continues next page

Drug	Nutritional Side Effects	Nutrition Plan (continued)
Tacrolimus (FK-506) (Prograf)[m]	• Hyperglycemia, glucose intolerance • Hyperlipidemia • Nausea/vomiting • Diarrhea • Abdominal gas/pain • Hyperkalemia • Hypokalemia • Hypomagnesemia • Hypophosphatemia • Hypertension, edema • Increased bone resorption	• Monitor blood sugar, may need to limit carbohydrates. • Reduce fat intake. • Monitor for adequate intake, try antiemetic medications. • Review drugs and consider a substitute for those that may be causing diarrhea, monitor and replace fluids as needed. • Monitor for adequate intake. • Restrict potassium intake. • Supplement with potassium-rich foods or supplements. • Supplement with magnesium-rich foods or supplements. • Supplement with phosphorus-rich foods or supplements. • Restrict sodium intake. • Monitor calcium and phosphorus levels; ensure adequate calcium and vitamin D intake; consider need for calcitonin, hormonal replacement, bisphosphonates.
Muromonab-CD3 (Orthoclone OKT3)[n]	• Nausea/vomiting • Diarrhea • Anorexia • Abdominal pain • Hypertension, edema • Hypotension • Fever	• Monitor for adequate intake, try antiemetic medications. • Review drugs and consider a substitute for those that may be causing diarrhea, monitor and replace fluids as needed. • Monitor for adequate intake, suggest frequent small meals. • Monitor for adequate intake. • Restrict sodium intake. • Maintain adequate fluid status. • Monitor dietary and fluid intake.
Basiliximab (Simulect)[a]	• Hyperglycemia, glucose intolerance • Hypercholesterolemia • Nausea/vomiting • Diarrhea • Abdominal pain • Hyperkalemia • Hypokalemia • Hypertension, edema • Fever	• Monitor blood sugar, may need to limit carbohydrates. • Reduce fat and cholesterol intake. • Monitor for adequate intake, try antiemetic medications. • Review drugs and consider a substitute for those that may be causing diarrhea, monitor and replace fluids as needed. • Monitor for adequate intake. • Restrict potassium intake. • Supplement with potassium-rich foods or supplements. • Restrict sodium intake. • Monitor dietary and fluid intake.
Daclizumab (Zenapax)[c]	• Hyperglycemia, glucose intolerance • Nausea/vomiting • Diarrhea • Abdominal pain • Hypertension, edema, fluid overload • Hypotension, dehydration • Fever	• Monitor blood sugar, may need to limit carbohydrates. • Monitor for adequate intake, try antiemetic medications. • Review drugs and consider a substitute for those that may be causing diarrhea, monitor and replace fluids as needed. • Monitor for adequate intake. • Restrict sodium intake. • Maintain adequate fluid status. • Monitor dietary and fluid intake.

[a]Novartis Pharmaceutical Corp, East Hanover, NJ 07936
[b]Abbott Laboratories, Abbott Park, IL 60064
[c]Hoffmann-La Roche, Inc, Nutley, NJ 07110
[d]Pharmacia and Upjohn Co, Kalamazoo, MI 49001
[e]Schering-Plough Corp, Kenilworth, NJ 07033
[f]Solvay Pharmaceuticals, Inc, Marietta, GA 30062

[g]Merz Pharmaceuticals, LLC, Greensboro, NC 27410
[h]Prometheus Laboratories Inc, San Diego, CA 92121
[j]SangStat Medical Corp, Fremont, CA 94555
[k]Wyeth Pharmaceuticals, Inc, St. Davids, PA 19087
[m]Fujisawa Healthcare, Inc, Deerfield, IL 60015
[n]Ortho Biotech, Inc, Raritan, NJ 08869

Bibliography

Byham Gray L. Nutritional implications of renal transplantation. *Renal Nutr Forum.* 1994;13:1–3.

Drug Facts and Comparisons. St Louis, Mo: Facts and Comparisons; 2002.

Epstein S, Shane E, Bilezikian JP. Organ transplantation and osteoporosis. *Curr Opin Rheumatol.* 1995;7:255–261.

First MR. An update on new immunosuppressive drugs undergoing preclinical and clinical trials: potential applications in organ transplantation. *Am J Kidney Dis.* 1997;29:303–317.

Hasse J. Nutritional management of renal transplant patients. *Dietetic Currents.* 1993;20(5):21–24.

Kopple JD, Massry SG, eds. *Nutritional Management of Renal Disease.* Baltimore, Md: Williams & Wilkins; 1997.

Matarese LE, Gottschlich MM. *Contemporary Nutrition Support Practice: A Clinical Guide.* Philadelphia, Pa: WB Saunders; 1998.

Moe SM. The treatment of steroid-induced bone loss in transplantation. *Curr Opin Nephrol Hypertens.* 1997; 6:544–549.

Physician's Desk Reference. 56th ed. Montvale, NJ: Medical Economics Co; 2002.

Strejc J, Weil S. Nutritional management of the renal transplant recipient. *Clin Strategies.* 1996;3(2):5,10,13.

INDEX